HEALTH PROFESSIONS:
DESCRIPTIONS AND INDEXES

HEALTH PROFESSIONS: DESCRIPTIONS AND INDEXES

JON V. HARRIS (EDITOR)

Novinka Books
New York

Senior Editors: Susan Boriotti and Donna Dennis
Coordinating Editor: Tatiana Shohov
Office Manager: Annette Hellinger
Graphics: Wanda Serrano
Editorial Production: Jennifer Vogt, Matthew Kozlowski, Jonathan Rose
and Maya Columbus
Circulation: Ave Maria Gonzalez, Vera Popovic, Luis Aviles, Melissa Diaz,
Vladimir Klestov and Jeannie Pappas
Communications and Acquisitions: Serge P. Shohov
Marketing: Cathy DeGregory

Library of Congress Cataloging-in-Publication Data
Available Upon Request

ISBN: 1-59033-465-5.

Copyright © 2002 by Novinka Books, An Imprint of
Nova Science Publishers, Inc.
400 Oser Ave, Suite 1600
Hauppauge, New York 11788-3619
Tele. 631-231-7269   Fax 631-231-8175
e-mail: Novascience@earthlink.net
Web Site: http://www.novapublishers.com

All rights reserved. No part of this book may be reproduced, stored in a retrieval system or transmitted in any form or by any means: electronic, electrostatic, magnetic, tape, mechanical photocopying, recording or otherwise without permission from the publishers.

The publisher has taken reasonable care in the preparation of this book, but makes no expressed or implied warranty of any kind and assumes no responsibility for any errors or omissions. No liability is assumed for incidental or consequential damages in connection with or arising out of information contained in this book.

This publication is designed to provide accurate and authoritative information with regard to the subject matter covered herein. It is sold with the clear understanding that the publisher is not engaged in rendering legal or any other professional services. If legal or any other expert assistance is required, the services of a competent person should be sought. FROM A DECLARATION OF PARTICIPANTS JOINTLY ADOPTED BY A COMMITTEE OF THE AMERICAN BAR ASSOCIATION AND A COMMITTEE OF PUBLISHERS.

Printed in the United States of America

Contents

Preface		vii
Chapter 1	Chiropractors	1
Chapter 2	Dentists	7
Chapter 3	Dietitians and Nutritionists	13
Chapter 4	Occupational Therapists	19
Chapter 5	Optometrists	25
Chapter 6	Pharmacists	31
Chapter 7	Physical Therapists	39
Chapter 8	Physician Assistants	45
Chapter 9	Physicians and Surgeons	51
Chapter 10	Podiatrists	59
Chapter 11	Recreational Therapists	65
Chapter 12	Registered Nurses	71
Chapter 13	Respiratory Therapists	79
Chapter 14	Speech-Language Pathologists and Audiologists	85
Chapter 15	Veterinarians	93
Chapter 16	Cardiovascular Technologists and Technicians	101
Chapter 17	Clinical Laboratory Technologists and Technicians	107

Chapter 18	Dental Hygienists	115
Chapter 19	Diagnostic Medical Sonographers	121
Chapter 20	Emergency Medical Technicians and Paramedics	127
Chapter 21	Licensed Practical and Licensed Vocational Nurses	135
Chapter 22	Medical Records and Health Information Technicians	141
Chapter 23	Nuclear Medicine Technologists	147
Chapter 24	Occupational Health and Safety Specialists and Technicians	153
Chapter 25	Opticians, Dispensing	161
Chapter 26	Pharmacy Technicians	167
Chapter 27	Radiologic Technologists and Technicians	173
Chapter 28	Surgical Technologists	179
Index		185

PREFACE

Maintaining one's bodily health is paramount toward having a satisfactory life. Health professionals, therefore, hold a key place in society. This book provides an overview of the different areas of work in the medical field, from ophthalmologists to podiatrists – head to toes and everything in between. Included in the descriptions are job qualifications and prospects, working conditions, and earnings. This book is a must to anyone considering entering this ever-growing occupation.

Chapter 1

CHIROPRACTORS

SIGNIFICANT POINTS

- Employment of chiropractors is expected to increase faster than average, and job prospects should be good.
- Chiropractic care of back, neck, extremities, and other joint damage has become more accepted as a result of recent research and changing attitudes.
- In chiropractic, as in other types of independent practice, earnings are relatively low in the beginning, but increase as the practice grows.

NATURE OF THE WORK

Chiropractors, also known as doctors of chiropractic or chiropractic physicians, diagnose and treat patients whose health problems are associated with the body's muscular, nervous, and skeletal systems, especially the spine. Chiropractors believe interference with these systems impairs normal functions and lowers resistance to disease. They also hold that spinal or vertebral dysfunction alters many important body functions by affecting the nervous system, and that skeletal imbalance through joint or articular dysfunction, especially in the spine, can cause pain.

The chiropractic approach to healthcare is holistic, stressing the patient's overall health and wellness. It recognizes that many factors affect health, including exercise, diet, rest, environment, and heredity. Chiropractors provide natural, drugless, nonsurgical health treatments, and rely on the body's inherent recuperative abilities. They also recommend lifestyle changes-in eating, exercise, and sleeping habits, for example-to their patients. When appropriate, chiropractors consult with and refer patients to other health practitioners.

Like other health practitioners, chiropractors follow a standard routine to secure the information needed for diagnosis and treatment. They take the patient's medical history, conduct physical, neurological, and orthopedic examinations, and may order laboratory tests. X rays and other diagnostic images are important tools because of the emphasis on the spine and its proper function. Chiropractors also employ a postural and spinal analysis common to chiropractic diagnosis.

In cases in which difficulties can be traced to involvement of musculoskeletal structures, chiropractors manually adjust the spinal column. Some chiropractors use water, light, massage, ultrasound, electric, and heat therapy. They also may apply supports such as straps, tapes, and braces. Chiropractors counsel patients about wellness concepts such as nutrition, exercise, lifestyle changes, and stress management, but do not prescribe drugs or perform surgery.

Some chiropractors specialize in sports injuries, neurology, orthopedics, pediatrics, nutrition, internal disorders, or diagnostic imaging.

Many chiropractors are solo or group practitioners who also have the administrative responsibilities of running a practice. In larger offices, chiropractors delegate these tasks to office managers and chiropractic assistants. Chiropractors in private practice are responsible for developing a patient base, hiring employees, and keeping records.

WORKING CONDITIONS

Chiropractors work in clean, comfortable offices. The average workweek is about 40 hours, although longer hours are not uncommon. Solo practitioners set their own hours, but may work evenings or weekends to accommodate patients.

Chiropractors, like other health practitioners, are sometimes on their feet for long periods. Chiropractors who take x rays must employ appropriate precautions against the dangers of repeated exposure to radiation.

EMPLOYMENT

Chiropractors held about 50,000 jobs in 2000. Most chiropractors are in solo practice, although some are in group practice or work for other chiropractors. A small number teach, conduct research at chiropractic institutions, or work in hospitals and clinics.

Many chiropractors are located in small communities. There are geographic imbalances in the distribution of chiropractors, in part because many establish practices close to chiropractic institutions.

TRAINING, OTHER QUALIFICATIONS AND ADVANCEMENT

All States and the District of Columbia regulate the practice of chiropractic and grant licenses to chiropractors who meet educational and examination requirements established by the State. Chiropractors can only practice in States where they are licensed. Some States have agreements permitting chiropractors licensed in one State to obtain a license in another without further examination, provided that educational, examination, and practice credentials meet State specifications. Most State boards require at least 2 years of undergraduate education, and an increasing number require a 4-year bachelor's degree. All boards require completion of a 4-year chiropractic college course at an accredited program leading to the Doctor of Chiropractic degree.

For licensure, most State boards recognize either all or part of the four-part test administered by the National Board of Chiropractic Examiners. State examinations may supplement the National Board tests, depending on State requirements.

To maintain licensure, almost all States require completion of a specified number of hours of continuing education each year. Continuing education programs are offered by accredited chiropractic programs and institutions, and chiropractic associations. Specialty councils within some chiropractic associations also offer programs leading to clinical specialty certification, called "diplomate" certification, in areas such as orthopedics, neurology, sports injuries, occupational and industrial health, nutrition, diagnostic imaging, thermography, and internal disorders.

In 2000, there were 16 chiropractic programs and institutions in the United States accredited by the Council on Chiropractic Education. All required applicants to have at least 60 semester hours of undergraduate study leading toward a bachelor's degree, including courses in English, the social sciences or humanities, organic and inorganic chemistry, biology, physics, and psychology. Many applicants have a bachelor's degree, which may eventually become the minimum entry requirement. Several chiropractic colleges offer prechiropractic study, as well as a bachelor's degree program. Recognition of prechiropractic education offered by chiropractic colleges varies among the State boards.

During the first 2 years, most chiropractic programs emphasize classroom and laboratory work in basic science subjects such as anatomy, physiology, public health, microbiology, pathology, and biochemistry. The last 2 years stress courses in manipulation and spinal adjustments, and provide clinical experience in physical and laboratory diagnosis, neurology, orthopedics, geriatrics, physiotherapy, and nutrition. Chiropractic programs and institutions grant the degree of Doctor of Chiropractic (DC). Chiropractic requires keen observation to detect physical abnormalities. It also takes considerable hand dexterity to perform adjustments, but not unusual strength or endurance. Chiropractors should be able to work independently and handle responsibility. As in other health-related occupations, empathy, understanding, and the desire to help others are good qualities for dealing effectively with patients.

Newly licensed chiropractors can set up a new practice, purchase an established one, or enter into partnership with an established practitioner. They also may take a salaried position with an established chiropractor, a group practice, or a healthcare facility.

JOB OUTLOOK

Job prospects are expected to be good for persons who enter the practice of chiropractic. Employment of chiropractors is expected to grow faster than the average for all occupations through the year 2010 as consumer demand for alternative healthcare grows. Chiropractors emphasize the importance of healthy lifestyles and do not prescribe drugs or perform surgery. As a result, chiropractic care is appealing to many health-conscious Americans. Chiropractic treatment of back, neck, extremities, and other joint damage has become more accepted as a result of recent research and changing attitudes about alternative healthcare practices. The rapidly expanding older population, with their increased likelihood of mechanical and structural problems, also will increase demand.

Demand for chiropractic treatment is also related to the ability of patients to pay, either directly or through health insurance. Although more insurance plans now cover chiropractic services, the extent of such coverage varies among plans. Increasingly, chiropractors must educate communities about the benefits of chiropractic care in order to establish a successful practice.

In this occupation, replacement needs arise almost entirely from retirements. Chiropractors usually remain in the occupation until they retire; few transfer to other occupations. Establishing a new practice will be easiest in areas with a low concentration of chiropractors.

EARNINGS

Median annual earnings of salaried chiropractors were $67,030 in 2000. The middle 50 percent earned between $44,030 and $105,520 a year.

Self-employed chiropractors usually earn more than salaried chiropractors. According to the American Chiropractic Association, in 2000, the average income for all chiropractors, including the self-employed, was about $81,500 after expenses. In chiropractic, as in other types of independent practice, earnings are relatively low in the beginning, and increase as the practice grows. Earnings also are influenced by the characteristics and qualifications of the practitioner, and geographic location. Self-employed chiropractors must provide for their own health insurance and retirement.

RELATED OCCUPATIONS

Chiropractors treat and work to prevent bodily disorders and injuries. So do dentists, occupational therapists, optometrists, physical therapists, physicians and surgeons, podiatrists, and veterinarians.

SOURCES OF ADDITIONAL INFORMATION

General information on chiropractic as a career is available from:

- American Chiropractic Association, 1701 Clarendon Blvd., Arlington, VA 22209. Internet: http://www.amerchiro.org
- International Chiropractors Association, 1110 North Glebe Rd., Suite 1000, Arlington, VA 22201. Internet: http://www.chiropractic.org
- World Chiropractic Alliance, 2950 N. Dobson Rd., Suite 1, Chandler, AZ 85224-1802. Internet: http://www.worldchiropracticalliance.org
- Dynamic Chiropractic, P.O. Box 40109, Huntington, CA 92605. Internet: http://www.chiroweb.com

For a list of chiropractic programs and institutions, as well as general information on chiropractic education, contact: Council on Chiropractic Education, 7975 North Hayden Rd., Suite A-210, Scottsdale, AZ 85258.

For information on State education and licensure requirements, contact: Federation of Chiropractic Licensing Boards, 901 54th Ave., Suite 101, Greeley, CO 80634. Internet: http://www.fclb.org/fclb

For information on requirements for admission to a specific chiropractic college, as well as scholarship and loan information, contact the admissions office of the individual college.

Chapter 2

DENTISTS

SIGNIFICANT POINTS

- Most dentists have at least 8 years of education beyond high school.
- Although employment growth will provide some job opportunities, most jobs will result from the need to replace the large number of dentists projected to retire.
- Dental care will increasingly focus on prevention, which involves teaching people how better to care for their teeth.

NATURE OF THE WORK

Dentists diagnose, prevent, and treat teeth and tissue problems. They remove decay, fill cavities, examine x-rays, place protective plastic sealants on children's teeth, straighten teeth, and repair fractured teeth. They also perform corrective surgery on gums and supporting bones to treat gum diseases. Dentists extract teeth and make models and measurements for dentures to replace missing teeth. They provide instruction on diet, brushing, flossing, use of fluorides, and other aspects of dental care, as well. They also administer anesthetics and write prescriptions for antibiotics and other medications. Dentists use a variety of equipment, including x-ray machines, drills, and instruments such as mouth mirrors, probes, forceps, brushes, and scalpels. They wear masks, gloves, and safety glasses to protect themselves and their patients from infectious diseases. Dentists in private practice oversee a variety of administrative tasks, including bookkeeping, and buying equipment and supplies. They may employ and supervise dental hygienists, dental assistants, dental laboratory technicians, and receptionists. Most dentists are general practitioners, handling a variety of dental needs. Other dentists practice in 1 of 9 specialty areas. Orthodontists, the largest group of specialists, straighten teeth by applying pressure to the teeth with braces or retainers. The next largest group, oral and maxillofacial surgeons, operate on the mouth and jaws. The remainder may specialize as pediatric dentists (focusing on dentistry for children); periodontists (treating gums and bone supporting the teeth); prosthodontists (replacing missing teeth with permanent fixtures, such as crowns and bridges, or removable fixtures, such as dentures); endodontists (performing root canal therapy); public health dentists (promoting good dental health and preventing dental diseases within the community); oral pathologists (studying oral diseases); or oral and maxillofacial radiologists (diagnosing diseases in the head and neck through the use of imaging technologies).

Working Conditions

Most dentists work 4 or 5 days a week. Some work evenings and weekends to meet their patients' needs. Most full-time dentists work about 40 hours a week, but others work more. Initially, dentists may work more hours as they establish their practice. Experienced dentists often work fewer hours. A considerable number continue in part-time practice well beyond the usual retirement age. Most dentists are "solo practitioners," meaning they own their own businesses and work alone or with a small staff. Some dentists have partners, and a few work for other dentists as associate dentists.

Employment

Dentists held about 152,000 jobs in 2000. Almost all dentists work in private practice. According to the American Dental Association, about 80 percent of dentists in private practice are sole proprietors, and 13 percent belong to a partnership. A small number of salaried dentists work in private or public hospitals and clinics.

TRAINING, OTHER QUALIFICATIONS AND ADVANCEMENT

All 50 States and the District of Columbia require dentists to be licensed. In most States, a candidate must graduate from a dental school accredited by the American Dental Association's Commission on Dental Accreditation, and pass written and practical examinations to qualify for a license. Candidates may fulfill the written part of the State licensing requirements by passing the National Board Dental Examinations. Individual States or regional testing agencies administer the written or practical examinations. Currently, about 17 States require dentists to obtain a specialty license before practicing as a specialist. Requirements include 2 to 4 years of postgraduate education and, in some cases, completion of a special State examination. Most State licenses permit dentists to engage in both general and specialized practice. Dentists who want to teach or do research usually spend an additional 2 to 5 years in advanced dental training, in programs operated by dental schools or hospitals. Dental schools require a minimum of 2 years of college-level predental education. However, most dental students have at least a bachelor's degree. Predental education emphasizes coursework in the sciences. All dental schools require applicants to take the Dental Admissions Test (DAT). When selecting students, schools consider scores earned on the DAT, applicants' grade point average, and information gathered through recommendations and interviews. Dental school usually lasts 4 academic years. Studies begin with classroom instruction and laboratory work in basic sciences, including anatomy, microbiology, biochemistry, and physiology. Beginning courses in clinical sciences, including laboratory techniques, also are provided at this time. During the last 2 years, students treat patients, usually in dental clinics, under the supervision of licensed dentists. Most dental schools award the degree of Doctor of Dental Surgery (DDS). The rest award an equivalent degree, Doctor of Dental Medicine (DMD).

Dentistry requires diagnostic ability and manual skills. Dentists should have good visual memory, excellent judgment of space and shape, a high degree of manual dexterity, and scientific ability. Good business sense, self-discipline, and communication skills are helpful for success in private practice. High school and college students who want to become dentists should take courses in biology, chemistry, physics, health, and mathematics. Some dental school graduates work for established dentists as associates for a year or two in order to gain experience and save money to equip an office of their own. Most dental school graduates, however, purchase an established practice or open a new one immediately after graduation. Each year, about one-fourth to one-third of new graduates enroll in postgraduate training programs to prepare for a dental specialty.

JOB OUTLOOK

Employment of dentists is expected to grow more slowly than the average for all occupations through 2010. Although employment growth will provide some job opportunities, most jobs will result from the need to replace the large number of dentists projected to retire. Job prospects should be good if the number of dental school graduates does not grow significantly, thus keeping the supply of newly qualified dentists near current levels. Demand for dental care should grow substantially through 2010. As members of the baby-boom generation advance into middle age, a large number will need maintenance on complicated dental work, such as bridges. In addition, elderly people are more likely to retain their teeth than were their predecessors, so they will require much more care than in the past. The younger generation will continue to need preventive checkups despite treatments such as fluoridation of the water supply, which decreases the incidence of tooth decay. Dental care will focus more on prevention, including teaching people how better to care for their teeth. Dentists will increasingly provide care that is aimed at preventing tooth loss-rather than simply providing treatments, such as fillings. Improvements in dental technology also will allow dentists to provide more effective and less painful treatment to their patients. However, the employment of dentists is not expected to grow as rapidly as the demand for dental services. As their practices expand, dentists are likely to hire more dental hygienists and dental assistants to handle routine services.

EARNINGS

Median annual earnings of salaried dentists were $129,030 in 2000. Earnings vary according to number of years in practice, location, hours worked, and specialty. Self-employed dentists in private practice tend to earn more than do salaried dentists. A relatively large proportion of dentists is self-employed. Like other business owners, these dentists must provide their own health insurance, life insurance, and retirement benefits.

RELATED OCCUPATIONS

Dentists examine, diagnose, prevent, and treat diseases and abnormalities. So do chiropractors, optometrists, physicians and surgeons, podiatrists, psychologists, and veterinarians.

SOURCES OF ADDITIONAL INFORMATION

For information on dentistry as a career and a list of accredited dental schools, contact: American Dental Association, Commission on Dental Accreditation, 211 E. Chicago Ave., Chicago, IL 60611. Internet: http://www.ada.org

For information on admission to dental schools, contact: American Dental Education Association, 1625 Massachusetts Ave. NW., Washington, DC 20036. Internet: http://www.adea.org

The American Dental Association also will furnish a list of State boards of dental examiners. Persons interested in practicing dentistry should obtain the requirements for licensure from the board of dental examiners of the State in which they plan to work. Prospective dental students should contact the office of student financial aid at the schools to which they apply, in order to obtain information on scholarships, grants, and loans, including Federal financial aid.

Chapter 3

DIETITIANS AND NUTRITIONISTS

SIGNIFICANT POINTS

- Employment of dietitians is expected to grow about as fast as the average for all occupations through the year 2010 as a result of increasing emphasis on disease prevention through improved health habits.
- Dietitians and nutritionists need at least a bachelor's degree in dietetics, foods and nutrition, food service systems management, or a related area.

NATURE OF THE WORK

Dietitians and nutritionists plan food and nutrition programs, and supervise the preparation and serving of meals. They help prevent and treat illnesses by promoting healthy eating habits and suggesting diet modifications, such as less salt for those with high blood pressure or reduced fat and sugar intake for those who are overweight.

Dietitians run food service systems for institutions such as hospitals and schools, promote sound eating habits through education, and conduct research. Major areas of practice include clinical, community, management, and consultant dietetics. Clinical dietitians provide nutritional services for patients in institutions such as hospitals and nursing homes. They assess patients' nutritional needs, develop and implement nutrition programs, and evaluate and report the results. They also confer with doctors and other healthcare professionals in order to coordinate medical and nutritional needs. Some clinical dietitians specialize in the management of overweight patients, care of the critically ill, or of renal (kidney) and diabetic patients. In addition, clinical dietitians in nursing homes, small hospitals, or correctional facilities also may manage the food service department.

Community dietitians counsel individuals and groups on nutritional practices designed to prevent disease and promote good health. Working in places such as public health clinics, home health agencies, and health maintenance organizations, they evaluate individual needs, develop nutritional care plans, and instruct individuals and their families. Dietitians working in home health agencies provide instruction on grocery shopping and food preparation to the elderly, individuals with special needs, and children. Increased interest in nutrition has led to opportunities in food manufacturing, advertising, and marketing, in which dietitians analyze foods, prepare literature for distribution, or report on issues such as the nutritional content of recipes, dietary fiber, or vitamin supplements.

Management dietitians oversee large-scale meal planning and preparation in healthcare facilities, company cafeterias, prisons, and schools. They hire, train, and direct other dietitians and food service workers; budget for and purchase food, equipment, and supplies; enforce sanitary and safety regulations; and prepare records and reports. Consultant dietitians work under contract with healthcare facilities or in their own private practice. They perform nutrition screenings for their clients, and offer advice on diet-related concerns such as weight loss or cholesterol reduction. Some work for wellness programs, sports teams, supermarkets, and other nutrition-related businesses. They may consult with food service managers, providing expertise in sanitation, safety procedures, menu development, budgeting, and planning.

WORKING CONDITIONS

Most dietitians work a regular 40-hour week, although some work weekends. Many dietitians work part time.

Dietitians and nutritionists usually work in clean, well-lighted, and well-ventilated areas. However, some dietitians work in warm, congested kitchens. Many dietitians and nutritionists are on their feet for much of the workday.

EMPLOYMENT

Dietitians and nutritionists held about 49,000 jobs in 2000. More than half were in hospitals, nursing homes, or offices and clinics of physicians.

State and local governments provided about 1 job in 10-mostly in health departments and other public health related areas. Other jobs were in restaurants, social service agencies, residential care facilities, diet workshops, physical fitness facilities, school systems, colleges and universities, and the Federal Government-mostly in the U.S. Department of Veterans Affairs. Some dietitians and nutritionists were employed by firms that provide food services on contract to such facilities as colleges and universities, airlines, correctional facilities, and company cafeterias.

Some dietitians were self-employed, working as consultants to facilities such as hospitals and nursing homes, or providing dietary counseling to individual clients.

TRAINING, OTHER QUALIFICATIONS AND ADVANCEMENT

High school students interested in becoming a dietitian or nutritionist should take courses in biology, chemistry, mathematics, health, and communications. Dietitians and nutritionists need at least a bachelor's degree in dietetics, foods and nutrition, food service systems management, or a related area. College students in these majors take courses in foods, nutrition, institution management, chemistry, biochemistry, biology, microbiology, and physiology. Other suggested courses include business, mathematics, statistics, computer science, psychology, sociology, and economics.

Twenty-seven of the 41 States with laws governing dietetics require licensure, 13 require certification, and 1 requires registration. The Commission on Dietetic Registration of the American Dietetic Association (ADA) awards the Registered Dietitian credential to those who pass a certification exam after completing their academic coursework and supervised experience. Because practice requirements vary by State, interested candidates should determine the requirements of the State in which they want to work before sitting for any exam.

As of 2001, there were 234 bachelor's and master's degree programs approved by the ADA's Commission on Accreditation for Dietetics Education (CADE). Supervised practice experience can be acquired in two ways. The first requires completion of an ADA-accredited coordinated program. As of 2001, there were 51 accredited programs, which combined academic and supervised practice experience and generally lasted 4 to 5 years. The second option requires completion of 900 hours of supervised practice experience in any of the 258 CADE-accredited/approved internships. Internships and may be full-time programs lasting 6 to 12 months, or part-time programs lasting 2 years. Students interested in research, advanced clinical positions, or public health may need an advanced degree.

Experienced dietitians may advance to assistant, associate, or director of a dietetic department, or become self-employed. Some dietitians specialize in areas such as renal or pediatric dietetics. Others may leave the occupation to become sales representatives for equipment, pharmaceutical, or food manufacturers.

JOB OUTLOOK

Employment of dietitians is expected to grow about as fast as the average for all occupations through 2010 as a result of increasing emphasis on disease prevention through improved dietary habits. A growing and aging population will increase the demand for meals and nutritional counseling in nursing homes, schools, prisons, community health programs, and home healthcare agencies. Public interest in nutrition and the emphasis on health education and prudent lifestyles will also spur demand, especially in management. In addition to employment growth, job openings also will result from the need to replace experienced workers who leave the occupation.

The number of dietitian positions in hospitals is expected to grow slowly as hospitals continue to contract out food service operations. On the other hand, employment is expected to grow fast in contract providers of food services, social service agencies, and offices and clinics of physicians. Employment growth for dietitians and nutritionists may be somewhat constrained by some employers substituting other workers such as health educators, food service managers, and dietetic technicians. Growth also is constrained by limitations on insurance reimbursement for dietetic services.

EARNINGS

Median annual earnings of dietitians and nutritionists were $38,450 in 2000. The middle 50 percent earned between $31,070 and $45,950 a year. The lowest 10 percent earned less than $23,680, and the highest 10 percent earned more than $54,940 a year. Median annual earnings in hospitals, the industry employing the largest numbers of dietitians and nutritionists, were $39,450.

According to the American Dietetic Association, median annual income for registered dietitians in 1999 varied by practice area as follows:

- $48,810 in consultation and business
- $48,370 in food and nutrition management
- $47,040 in education and research
- $37,990 in community nutrition, and
- $37,565 in clinical nutrition.

Salaries also vary by years in practice, educational level, geographic region, and size of community.

RELATED OCCUPATIONS

Workers in other occupations who may apply the principles of food and nutrition include food service managers, health educators, and registered nurses.

SOURCES OF ADDITIONAL INFORMATION

For a list of academic programs, scholarships, and other information about dietetics, contact: The American Dietetic Association, 216 West Jackson Blvd., Suite 800, Chicago, IL 60606-6995. Internet: http://www.eatright.org

Chapter 4

OCCUPATIONAL THERAPISTS

SIGNIFICANT POINTS

- Employment is projected to increase faster than the average, as rapid growth in the number of middle-aged and elderly individuals increases the demand for therapeutic services.
- Occupational therapists are increasingly taking on supervisory roles.
- More than one-third of occupational therapists work part time.

NATURE OF THE WORK

Occupational therapists (OTs) help people improve their ability to perform tasks in their daily living and working environments. They work with individuals who have conditions that are mentally, physically, developmentally, or emotionally disabling. They also help them to develop, recover, or maintain daily living and work skills. Occupational therapists not only help clients improve basic motor functions and reasoning abilities, but also compensate for permanent loss of function. Their goal is to help clients have independent, productive, and satisfying lives.

Occupational therapists assist clients in performing activities of all types, ranging from using a computer, to caring for daily needs such as dressing, cooking, and eating. Physical exercises may be used to increase strength and dexterity, while paper and pencil exercises may be chosen to improve visual acuity and the ability to discern patterns. A client with short-term memory loss, for instance, might be encouraged to make lists to aid recall. A person with coordination problems might be assigned exercises to improve hand-eye coordination. Occupational therapists also use computer programs to help clients improve decision making, abstract reasoning, problem solving, and perceptual skills, as well as memory, sequencing, and coordination-all of which are important for independent living.

For those with permanent functional disabilities, such as spinal cord injuries, cerebral palsy, or muscular dystrophy, therapists instruct in the use of adaptive equipment such as wheelchairs, splints, and aids for eating and dressing. They also design or make special equipment needed at home or at work. Therapists develop computer-aided adaptive equipment and teach clients with severe limitations how to use it. This equipment enables clients to communicate better and to control other aspects of their environment.

Some occupational therapists, called industrial therapists, treat individuals whose ability to function in a work environment has been impaired. They arrange employment, plan work activities, and evaluate the client's progress.

Occupational therapists may work exclusively with individuals in a particular age group, or with particular disabilities. In schools, for example, they evaluate children's abilities, recommend and provide therapy, modify classroom equipment, and in general, help children participate as fully as possible in school programs and activities. Occupational therapy is also beneficial to the elderly population. Therapists help senior citizens lead more productive, active and independent lives through a variety of methods, including the use of adaptive equipment.

Occupational therapists in mental health settings treat individuals who are mentally ill, mentally retarded, or emotionally disturbed. To treat these problems, therapists choose activities that help people learn to cope with daily life. Activities include time management skills, budgeting, shopping, homemaking, and use of public transportation. They may also work with individuals who are dealing with alcoholism, drug abuse, depression, eating disorders, or stress related disorders.

Recording a client's activities and progress is an important part of an occupational therapist's job. Accurate records are essential for evaluating clients, billing, and reporting to physicians and others.

WORKING CONDITIONS

Occupational therapists in hospitals and other health care and community settings usually work a 40-hour week. Those in schools may also participate in meetings and other activities, during and after the school day. More than one-third of occupational therapists work part time.

In large rehabilitation centers, therapists may work in spacious rooms equipped with machines, tools, and other devices generating noise. The job can be tiring, because therapists are on their feet much of the time. Those providing home healthcare may spend time driving from appointment to appointment. Therapists also face hazards such as back strain from lifting and moving clients and equipment.

Therapists are increasingly taking on supervisory roles. Due to rising healthcare costs, third party payers are beginning to encourage occupational therapist assistants and aides to take more hands-on responsibility. By having assistants and aides work more closely with clients under the guidance of a therapist, the cost of therapy should be more modest.

EMPLOYMENT

Occupational therapists held about 78,000 jobs in 2000. About 1 in 6 occupational therapists held more than one job in 2000. The largest number of jobs was in hospitals, including many in rehabilitation and psychiatric hospitals. Other major employers include offices and clinics of occupational therapists and other health practitioners, school systems, home health agencies, nursing homes, community mental health centers, adult daycare programs, job training services, and residential care facilities.

Some occupational therapists are self-employed in private practice. They see clients referred by physicians or other health professionals, or provide contract or consulting services to nursing homes, schools, adult daycare programs, and home health agencies.

Training, Other Qualifications and Advancement

A bachelor's degree in occupational therapy is the minimum requirement for entry into this field. All States, Puerto Rico, and the District of Columbia regulate occupational therapy. To obtain a license, applicants must graduate from an accredited educational program, and pass a national certification examination. Those who pass the test are awarded the title of registered occupational therapist.

In 1999, entry-level education was offered in 88 bachelor's degree programs; 11 postbachelor's certificate programs for students with a degree other than occupational therapy; and 53 entry-level master's degree programs. Nineteen programs offered a combined bachelor's and master's degree and 2 offered an entry-level doctoral degree. Most schools have full-time programs, although a growing number also offer weekend or part-time programs.

Occupational therapy coursework includes physical, biological, and behavioral sciences, and the application of occupational therapy theory and skills. Completion of 6 months of supervised fieldwork also is required.

Persons considering this profession should take high school courses in biology, chemistry, physics, health, art, and the social sciences. College admissions offices also look favorably at paid or volunteer experience in the healthcare field.

Occupational therapists need patience and strong interpersonal skills to inspire trust and respect in their clients. Ingenuity and imagination in adapting activities to individual needs are assets. Those working in home healthcare must be able to successfully adapt to a variety of settings.

Job Outlook

Employment of occupational therapists is expected to increase faster than the average for all occupations through 2010. Federal legislation imposing limits on reimbursement for therapy services may adversely affect the job market for occupational therapists in the near term. However, over the long run, the demand for occupational therapists should continue to rise as a result of growth in the number of individuals with disabilities or limited function requiring therapy services. The baby-boom generation's movement into middle age, a period when the incidence of heart attack and stroke increases, will increase the demand for therapeutic services. The rapidly growing population 75 years of age and above (an age that suffers from a high incidence of disabling conditions), also will demand additional services. Medical advances now enable more patients with critical problems to survive. These patients may need extensive therapy. Hospitals will continue to employ a large number of occupational therapists to provide therapy services to acutely ill inpatients. Hospitals will also need occupational therapists to staff their outpatient rehabilitation programs. Employment growth in schools will result from expansion of the school-age population and extended services for disabled students. Therapists will be needed to help children with disabilities prepare to enter special education programs.

EARNINGS

Median annual earnings of occupational therapists were $49,450 in 2000. The middle 50 percent earned between $40,460 and $57,890. The lowest 10 percent earned less than $32,040, and the highest 10 percent earned more than $70,810. Median annual earnings in the industries employing the largest numbers of occupational therapists in 2000 were as follows:

- Nursing and personal care facilities $51,220
- Hospitals $50,430
- Offices of other health practitioners $49,520
- Elementary and secondary schools $45,340

RELATED OCCUPATIONS

Occupational therapists use specialized knowledge to help individuals perform daily living skills and achieve maximum independence. Other workers performing similar duties include chiropractors, physical therapists, recreational therapists, rehabilitation counselors, respiratory therapists, and speech-language pathologists and audiologists.

SOURCES OF ADDITIONAL INFORMATION

For more information on occupational therapy as a career, contact:

- The American Occupational Therapy Association, 4720 Montgomery Lane, P.O. Box 31220, Bethesda, MD 20824-1220. Internet: http://www.aota.org

Chapter 5

OPTOMETRISTS

SIGNIFICANT POINTS

- Licensed optometrists must earn a Doctor of Optometry degree from an accredited optometry school and pass a written and a clinical State board examination.
- Competition for admission to optometry school is keen.
- Because optometrists usually remain in practice until they retire, replacement needs arise almost entirely from retirements.

NATURE OF THE WORK

More than half of the people in the United States wear glasses or contact lenses. Optometrists, also known as doctors of optometry, or ODs, provide most primary vision care.

Optometrists examine people's eyes to diagnose vision problems and eye diseases. They use instruments and observation to examine eye health and to test patients' visual acuity, depth and color perception, and ability to focus and coordinate the eyes. Optometrists analyze test results and develop a treatment plan. Optometrists prescribe eyeglasses and contact lenses, and provide vision therapy and low vision rehabilitation. They administer drugs to patients to aid in the diagnosis of eye vision problems and prescribe drugs to treat some eye diseases. Optometrists often provide preoperative and postoperative care to cataract, laser vision correction, and other eye surgery patients. They also diagnose conditions due to systemic diseases such as diabetes and high blood pressure, and refer patients to other health practitioners as needed.

Optometrists should not be confused with ophthalmologists or dispensing opticians. Ophthalmologists are physicians who perform eye surgery, and diagnose and treat eye diseases and injuries. Like optometrists, they also examine eyes and prescribe eyeglasses and contact lenses. Dispensing opticians fit and adjust eyeglasses and in some States may fit contact lenses according to prescriptions written by ophthalmologists or optometrists. Most optometrists are in general practice. Some specialize in work with the elderly, children, or partially sighted persons who need specialized visual devices. Others develop and implement ways to protect workers' eyes from on-the-job strain or injury. Some specialize in contact lenses, sports vision, or vision therapy. A few teach optometry, perform research, or consult.

Most optometrists are private practitioners who also handle the business aspects of running an office, such as developing a patient base, hiring employees, keeping records, and ordering equipment and supplies. Optometrists who operate franchise optical stores also may have some of these duties.

WORKING CONDITIONS

Optometrists work in places-usually their own offices-which are clean, well-lighted, and comfortable. Most full-time optometrists work about 40 hours a week. Many work Saturdays and evenings to suit the needs of patients. Emergency calls, once uncommon, have increased with the passage of therapeutic drug laws expanding optometrists' ability to prescribe medications.

EMPLOYMENT

Optometrists held about 31,000 jobs in 2000. The number of jobs is greater than the number of practicing optometrists because some optometrists hold two or more jobs. For example, an optometrist may have a private practice, but also work in another practice, clinic, or vision care center. According to the American Optometric Association, about two-thirds of practicing optometrists are in private practice.

Although many optometrists practice alone, a growing number are in a partnership or group practice. Some optometrists work as salaried employees of other optometrists or of ophthalmologists, hospitals, health maintenance organizations (HMOs), or retail optical stores. A small number of optometrists are consultants for industrial safety programs, insurance companies, manufacturers of ophthalmic products, HMOs, and others.

TRAINING, OTHER QUALIFICATIONS AND ADVANCEMENT

All States and the District of Columbia require that optometrists be licensed. Applicants for a license must have a Doctor of Optometry degree from an accredited optometry school and pass both a written and a clinical State board examination. In many States, applicants can substitute the examinations of the National Board of Examiners in Optometry, usually taken during the student's academic career, for part or all of the written examination. Licenses are renewed every 1 to 3 years and in all States, continuing education credits are needed for renewal.

The Doctor of Optometry degree requires completion of a 4-year program at an accredited optometry school preceded by at least 3 years of preoptometric study at an accredited college or university (most optometry students hold a bachelor's or higher degree). In 2000, 17 U.S. schools and colleges of optometry held an accredited status with the Accreditation Council on Optometric Education of the American Optometric Association.

Requirements for admission to schools of optometry include courses in English, mathematics, physics, chemistry, and biology. A few schools require or recommend courses in psychology, history, sociology, speech, or business. Applicants must take the Optometry Admissions Test, which measures academic ability and scientific comprehension. Most applicants take the test after their sophomore or junior year. Competition for admission is keen.

Optometry programs include classroom and laboratory study of health and visual sciences, as well as clinical training in the diagnosis and treatment of eye disorders. Courses in pharmacology, optics, vision science, biochemistry, and systemic disease are included.

Business ability, self-discipline, and the ability to deal tactfully with patients are important for success. The work of optometrists requires attention to detail and good manual dexterity.

Optometrists wishing to teach or do research may study for a master's or Ph.D. degree in visual science, physiological optics, neurophysiology, public health, health administration, health information and communication, or health education. One-year postgraduate clinical residency programs are available for optometrists who wish to specialize in family practice optometry, pediatric optometry, geriatric optometry, vision therapy, contact lenses, hospital-based optometry, primary care optometry, or ocular disease.

JOB OUTLOOK

Employment of optometrists is expected to grow about as fast as the average for all occupations through 2010 in response to the vision care needs of a growing and aging population. As baby boomers age, they will be more likely to visit optometrists and ophthalmologists because of the onset of vision problems in middle age, including those resulting from the extensive use of computers. The demand for optometric services also will increase because of growth in the oldest age group, with their increased likelihood of cataracts, glaucoma, diabetes, and hypertension. Employment of optometrists also will grow due to greater recognition of the importance of vision care, rising personal incomes, and growth in employee vision care plans. Employment of optometrists would grow more rapidly were it not for anticipated productivity gains that will allow each optometrist to see more patients. These expected gains stem from greater use of optometric assistants and other support personnel, who will reduce the amount of time optometrists need with each patient. Also, new surgical procedures using lasers are available that can correct some vision problems, but they remain expensive. Optometrists will still be needed to perform pre-operative and post-operative care for laser surgery; however, patients who successfully undergo this surgery may not require optometrists to prescribe glasses or contacts for several years.

In addition to growth, the need to replace optometrists who leave the occupation will create employment opportunities. Relatively few opportunities from this source are expected, however, because optometrists usually continue to practice until they retire; few transfer to other occupations.

EARNINGS

Median annual earnings of salaried optometrists were $82,860 in 2000. The middle 50 percent earned between $60,310 and $111,520. Median annual earnings of salaried optometrists in 2000 were $89,460 in offices and clinics of medical doctors and $85,470 in offices of other health practitioners. Salaried optometrists tend to earn more initially than do optometrists who set up their own independent practice. In the long run, those in private practice usually earn more.

According to the American Optometric Association, median net income for all optometrists in private practice ranged from about $115,000 to $120,000 in 2000.

RELATED OCCUPATIONS

Workers in other occupations who apply scientific knowledge to prevent, diagnose, and treat disorders and injuries are chiropractors, dentists, physicians and surgeons, podiatrists, speech-language pathologists and audiologists, and veterinarians.

SOURCES OF ADDITIONAL INFORMATION

For information on optometry as a career and a list of accredited optometric educational institutions, contact: Association of Schools and Colleges of Optometry, 6110 Executive Blvd., Suite 510, Rockville, MD 20852. Internet: http://www.opted.org

Additional career information is available from: American Optometric Association, Educational Services, 243 North Lindbergh Blvd., St. Louis, MO 63141-7881. Internet: http://www.aoanet.org

The Board of Optometry in each State can supply information on licensing requirements. For information on specific admission requirements and sources of financial aid, contact the admissions officer of individual optometry schools.

Chapter 6

PHARMACISTS

SIGNIFICANT POINTS

- Pharmacists are becoming more involved in drug therapy decision-making and patient counseling.
- A license is required; one must serve an internship under a licensed pharmacist, graduate from an accredited college of pharmacy, and pass a State examination.
- Very good employment opportunities are expected.
- Earnings are very high, but some pharmacists work long hours, nights, weekends, and holidays.

NATURE OF THE WORK

Pharmacists dispense drugs prescribed by physicians and other health practitioners and provide information to patients about medications and their use. They advise physicians and other health practitioners on the selection, dosages, interactions, and side effects of medications. Pharmacists must understand the use; clinical effects; and composition of drugs, including their chemical, biological, and physical properties. Compounding-the actual mixing of ingredients to form powders, tablets, capsules, ointments, and solutions-is only a small part of a pharmacist's practice, because most medicines are produced by pharmaceutical companies in a standard dosage and drug delivery form. Most pharmacists work either in a community setting, such as a retail drug store, or in a hospital or clinic.

Pharmacists in community or retail pharmacies counsel patients and answer questions about prescription drugs, such as those about possible adverse reactions or interactions. They provide information about over-the-counter drugs and make recommendations after asking a series of health questions, such as whether the customer is taking any other medications. They also give advice about durable medical equipment and home healthcare supplies. They also may complete third-party insurance forms and other paperwork. Those who own or manage community pharmacies may sell nonhealth-related merchandise, hire and supervise personnel, and oversee the general operation of the pharmacy. Some community pharmacists provide specialized services to help patients manage conditions such as diabetes, asthma, smoking cessation, or high blood pressure. Pharmacists in hospitals and clinics dispense medications and advise the medical staff on the selection and effects of drugs. They may make sterile solutions and buy medical supplies. They also assess, plan, and monitor drug programs or regimens. They counsel patients on the use of drugs while in the hospital, and on their use at home when the patients are discharged. Pharmacists also may evaluate drug use patterns and outcomes for patients in hospitals or managed care organizations.

Pharmacists who work in home healthcare monitor drug therapy and prepare infusions-solutions that are injected into patients-and other medications for use in the home.

Most pharmacists keep confidential computerized records of patients' drug therapies to ensure that harmful drug interactions do not occur. They frequently teach pharmacy students serving as interns in preparation for graduation and licensure.

Some pharmacists specialize in specific drug therapy areas, such as intravenous nutrition support, oncology (cancer), nuclear pharmacy (used for chemotherapy), and pharmacotherapy (the treatment of mental disorders with drugs).

Pharmacists are responsible for the accuracy of every prescription that is filled, but they often rely upon pharmacy technicians and pharmacy aides to assist them. Thus, the pharmacist may delegate prescription-filling and administrative tasks and supervise their completion.

Working Conditions

Pharmacists usually work in clean, well-lighted, and well-ventilated areas. Many pharmacists spend most of their workday on their feet. When working with sterile or potentially dangerous pharmaceutical products, pharmacists wear gloves and masks and work with other special protective equipment. Many community and hospital pharmacies are open for extended hours or around the clock, so pharmacists may work evenings, nights, weekends, and holidays. Consultant pharmacists may travel to nursing homes or other facilities to monitor patient's drug therapy.

About 1 out of 7 pharmacists worked part time in 2000. Most full-time salaried pharmacists worked about 40 hours a week. Some, including many self-employed pharmacists, worked more than 50 hours a week.

Employment

Pharmacists held about 217,000 jobs in 2000. About 6 out of 10 worked in community pharmacies, either independently owned or part of a drug store chain, grocery store, department store, or mass merchandiser. Most community pharmacists were salaried employees, but some were self-employed owners. About 21 percent of salaried pharmacists worked in hospitals, and others worked in clinics, mail-order pharmacies, pharmaceutical wholesalers, home healthcare agencies, or the Federal Government.

Training, Other Qualifications and Advancement

A license to practice pharmacy is required in all States, the District of Columbia, and U.S. territories. To obtain a license, one must serve an internship under a licensed pharmacist, graduate from an accredited college of pharmacy, and pass a State examination. All States, except California and Florida, currently grant a license without extensive re-examination to qualified pharmacists already licensed by another State; one should check with State boards of pharmacy for details. Many pharmacists are licensed to practice in more than one State. States may require continuing education for license renewal.

In 2000, 82 colleges of pharmacy were accredited to confer degrees by the American Council on Pharmaceutical Education. Pharmacy programs grant the degree of Doctor of Pharmacy (Pharm.D.), which requires at least 6 years of postsecondary study and the passing of the licensure examination of a State board of pharmacy. The Pharm.D. is a 4-year program that requires at least 2 years of college study prior to admittance. This degree has replaced the Bachelor of Science (B.S.) degree, which will cease to be awarded after 2005. Colleges of pharmacy require at least 2 years of college-level prepharmacy education. Entry requirements usually include mathematics and natural sciences, such as chemistry, biology, and physics, as well as courses in the humanities and social sciences. Some colleges require the applicant to take the Pharmacy College Admissions Test.

All colleges of pharmacy offer courses in pharmacy practice, designed to teach students to dispense prescriptions and to communicate with patients and other health professionals. Such courses also strengthen students' understanding of professional ethics and allow them to practice management responsibilities. Pharmacists' training increasingly emphasizes direct patient care, as well as consultative services to other health professionals.

In the 2000-01 academic year, 64 colleges of pharmacy awarded the master of science degree or the Ph.D. degree. Both the master's and Ph.D. degrees are awarded after completion of a Pharm.D. degree. These degrees are designed for those who want more laboratory and research experience. Many master's and Ph.D. holders work in research for a drug company or teach at a university. Other options for pharmacy graduates who are interested in further training include 1- or 2-year residency programs or fellowships. Pharmacy residencies are postgraduate training programs in pharmacy practice. Pharmacy fellowships are highly individualized programs designed to prepare participants to work in research laboratories. Some pharmacists who run their own pharmacy obtain a master's degree in business administration (MBA). Areas of graduate study include pharmaceutics and pharmaceutical chemistry (physical and chemical properties of drugs and dosage forms), pharmacology (effects of drugs on the body), and pharmacy administration.

Prospective pharmacists should have scientific aptitude, good communication skills, and a desire to help others. They also must be conscientious and pay close attention to detail, because the decisions they make affect human lives.

In community pharmacies, pharmacists usually begin at the staff level. After they gain experience and secure the necessary capital, some become owners or part owners of pharmacies. Pharmacists in chain drug stores may be promoted to pharmacy supervisor or manager at the store level, then to manager at the district or regional level, and later to an executive position within the chain's headquarters.

Hospital pharmacists may advance to supervisory or administrative positions. Pharmacists in the pharmaceutical industry may advance in marketing, sales, research, quality control, production, packaging, or other areas.

JOB OUTLOOK

Very good employment opportunities are expected for pharmacists over the 2000-10 period because the number of degrees granted in pharmacy are not expected to be as numerous as the number of job openings created by employment growth and the need to replace pharmacists who retire or otherwise leave the occupation.

Employment of pharmacists is expected to grow faster than the average for all occupations through the year 2010, due to the increased pharmaceutical needs of a larger and older population and greater use of medication. The growing numbers of middle-aged and elderly people-who, on average, use more prescription drugs than do younger people-will continue to spur demand for pharmacists in all practice settings. Other factors likely to increase the demand for pharmacists include scientific advances that will make more drug products available, new developments in genome research and medication distribution systems, and increasingly sophisticated consumers seeking more information about drugs.

Retail pharmacies are taking steps to increase their prescription volume to make up for declining dispensing fees. Automation of drug dispensing and greater use of pharmacy technicians and pharmacy aides will help them to dispense more prescriptions. The number of community pharmacists needed in the future will depend on the rate of expansion of chain drug stores and the willingness of insurers to reimburse pharmacists for providing clinical services to patients taking prescription medications. With its emphasis on cost control, managed care encourages growth of lower cost prescription drug distributors, such as mail-order firms, for certain medications. Faster than average employment growth is expected in retail pharmacies.

Employment in hospitals is expected to grow about as fast as average, as hospitals reduce inpatient stays, downsize, and consolidate departments. Pharmacy services are shifting to long-term, ambulatory, and home care settings, where opportunities for pharmacists will be best. New opportunities are emerging for pharmacists in managed-care organizations, where they may analyze trends and patterns in medication use for their populations of patients, and for pharmacists trained in research, disease management, and pharmacoeconomics-determining the costs and benefits of different drug therapies.

Cost-conscious insurers and health systems may continue to emphasize the role of pharmacists in primary and preventive health services. They realize that the expense of using medication to treat diseases and conditions often is considerably less than the potential costs for patients whose conditions go untreated. Pharmacists also can reduce the expenses resulting from unexpected complications due to allergic reactions or medication interactions.

EARNINGS

Median annual earnings of pharmacists in 2000 were $70,950. The middle 50 percent earned between $61,860 and $81,690 a year. The lowest 10 percent earned less than $51,570, and the highest 10 percent, more than $89,010 a year. Median annual earnings in the industries employing the largest numbers of pharmacists in 2000 were as follows:

- Department stores $73,730
- Grocery stores $72,440
- Drug stores and proprietary stores $72,110
- Hospitals $68,760

According to a survey by Drug Topics magazine, published by Medical Economics Co., average starting base salaries of full-time, salaried pharmacists were $67,824 in 2000. Pharmacists working in chain drug stores had an average annual base salary of $71,486 while pharmacists working in independent drug stores averaged $62,040 and hospital pharmacists averaged $61,250. Many pharmacists also receive compensation in the form of bonuses, overtime, and profit-sharing.

RELATED OCCUPATIONS

Pharmacy technicians and pharmacy aides also work in pharmacies. Persons in other professions who may work with pharmaceutical compounds include biological and medical scientists and chemists and materials scientists.

SOURCES OF ADDITIONAL INFORMATION

For information on pharmacy as a career, preprofessional and professional requirements, programs offered by colleges of pharmacy, and student financial aid, contact:

- American Association of Colleges of Pharmacy, 1426 Prince St., Alexandria, VA 22314. Internet: http://www.aacp.org
- National Association of Boards of Pharmacy, 700 Busse Highway, Park Ridge, IL 60068. Internet: http://www.nabp.net

General information on careers in pharmacy is available from: National Association of Chain Drug Stores, 413 N. Lee St., P.O. Box 1417-D49, Alexandria, VA 22313-1480. Internet: http://www.nacds.org

State licensure requirements are available from each State's Board of Pharmacy. Information on specific college entrance requirements, curriculums, and financial aid is available from any college of pharmacy.

Chapter 7

PHYSICAL THERAPISTS

SIGNIFICANT POINTS

- Employment is expected to increase faster than the average, as rapid growth in the number of middle-aged and elderly individuals increases the demand for therapeutic services.
- After graduating from an accredited physical therapist educational program, therapists must pass a licensure exam before they can practice.

NATURE OF THE WORK

Physical therapists (PTs) provide services that help restore function, improve mobility, relieve pain, and prevent or limit permanent physical disabilities of patients suffering from injuries or disease. They restore, maintain, and promote overall fitness and health. Their patients include accident victims and individuals with disabling conditions such as low back pain, arthritis, heart disease, fractures, head injuries, and cerebral palsy.

Therapists examine patients' medical histories, then test and measure their strength, range of motion, balance and coordination, posture, muscle performance, respiration, and motor function. They also determine patients' ability to be independent and reintegrate into the community or workplace after injury or illness. Next, they develop treatment plans describing a treatment strategy, its purpose, and anticipated outcome. Physical therapist assistants, under the direction and supervision of a physical therapist, may be involved in implementing treatment plans with patients. Physical therapist aides perform routine support tasks, as directed by the therapist. Treatment often includes exercise for patients who have been immobilized and lack flexibility, strength, or endurance. They encourage patients to use their own muscles to further increase flexibility and range of motion before finally advancing to other exercises improving strength, balance, coordination, and endurance. Their goal is to improve how an individual functions at work and home.

Physical therapists also use electrical stimulation, hot packs or cold compresses, and ultrasound to relieve pain and reduce swelling. They may use traction or deep-tissue massage to relieve pain. Therapists also teach patients to use assistive and adaptive devices such as crutches, prostheses, and wheelchairs. They also may show patients exercises to do at home to expedite their recovery. As treatment continues, physical therapists document progress, conduct periodic examinations, and modify treatments when necessary. Such documentation is used to track the patient's progress, and identify areas requiring more or less attention.

Physical therapists often consult and practice with a variety of other professionals, such as physicians, dentists, nurses, educators, social workers, occupational therapists, speech-language pathologists, and audiologists.

Some physical therapists treat a wide range of ailments; others specialize in areas such as pediatrics, geriatrics, orthopedics, sports medicine, neurology, and cardiopulmonary physical therapy.

Working Conditions

Physical therapists practice in hospitals, clinics, and private offices that have specially equipped facilities, or they treat patients in hospital rooms, homes, or schools.

Most full-time physical therapists work a 40-hour week, which may include some evenings and weekends. The job can be physically demanding because therapists often have to stoop, kneel, crouch, lift, and stand for long periods. In addition, physical therapists move heavy equipment and lift patients or help them turn, stand, or walk.

EMPLOYMENT

Physical therapists held about 132,000 jobs in 2000; about 1 in 4 worked part time. The number of jobs is greater than the number of practicing physical therapists because some physical therapists hold two or more jobs. For example, some may work in a private practice, but also work part time in another health facility.

About two-thirds of physical therapists were employed in either hospitals or offices of physical therapists. Other jobs were in home health agencies, outpatient rehabilitation centers, offices and clinics of physicians, and nursing homes. Some physical therapists are self-employed in private practices. They may provide services to individual patients or contract to provide services in hospitals, rehabilitation centers, nursing homes, home health agencies, adult daycare programs, and schools. They may be in solo practice or be part of a consulting group. Physical therapists also teach in academic institutions and conduct research.

TRAINING, OTHER QUALIFICATIONS AND ADVANCEMENT

All States require physical therapists to pass a licensure exam before they can practice, after graduating from an accredited physical therapist educational program.

According to the American Physical Therapy Association, there were 199 accredited physical therapist programs in 2001. Of the accredited programs, 165 offered master's degrees, and 33 offered doctoral degrees. By 2002, all physical therapist programs seeking accreditation are required to offer degrees at the master's degree level and above, in accordance with the Commission on Accreditation in Physical Therapy Education.

Physical therapist programs start with basic science courses such as biology, chemistry, and physics, and then introduce specialized courses such as biomechanics, neuroanatomy, human growth and development, manifestations of disease, examination techniques, and therapeutic procedures. Besides classroom and laboratory instruction, students receive supervised clinical experience. Courses useful when applying to physical therapist educational programs include anatomy, biology, chemistry, social science, mathematics, and physics. Before granting admission, many professional education programs require experience as a volunteer in a physical therapy department of a hospital or clinic.

Physical therapists should have strong interpersonal skills to successfully educate patients about their physical therapy treatments. They should also be compassionate and possess a desire to help patients. Similar traits also are needed to interact with the patient's family.

Physical therapists are expected to continue professional development by participating in continuing education courses and workshops. A number of States require continuing education to maintain licensure.

JOB OUTLOOK

Employment of physical therapists is expected to grow faster than the average for all occupations through 2010. Federal legislation imposing limits on reimbursement for therapy services may adversely affect the job market for physical therapists in the near term. However, over the long run, the demand for physical therapists should continue to rise as a result of growth in the number of individuals with disabilities or limited function requiring therapy services. The rapidly growing elderly population is particularly vulnerable to chronic and debilitating conditions that require therapeutic services. Also, the baby-boom generation is entering the prime age for heart attacks and strokes, increasing the demand for cardiac and physical rehabilitation. More young people will need physical therapy as technological advances save the lives of a larger proportion of newborns with severe birth defects.

Future medical developments should also permit a higher percentage of trauma victims to survive, creating additional demand for rehabilitative care. Growth also may result from advances in medical technology which permit treatment of more disabling conditions.

Widespread interest in health promotion also should increase demand for physical therapy services. A growing number of employers are using physical therapists to evaluate worksites, develop exercise programs, and teach safe work habits to employees in the hope of reducing injuries.

EARNINGS

Median annual earnings of physical therapists were $54,810 in 2000. The middle 50 percent earned between $46,660 and $67,390. The lowest 10 percent earned less than $38,510, and the highest 10 percent earned more than $83,370. Median annual earnings in the industries employing the largest numbers of physical therapists in 2000 were as follows:

- Offices and clinics of medical doctors $58,390
- Home health care services $57,830
- Offices of other health practitioners $55,830
- Nursing and personal care facilities $54,740
- Hospitals $54,430

RELATED OCCUPATIONS

Physical therapists rehabilitate persons with physical disabilities. Others who work in the rehabilitation field include occupational therapists, recreational therapists, rehabilitation counselors, respiratory therapists, and speech-language pathologists and audiologists.

SOURCES OF ADDITIONAL INFORMATION

Additional information on a career as a physical therapist and a list of accredited educational programs in physical therapy are available from: American Physical Therapy Association, 1111 North Fairfax St., Alexandria, VA 22314-1488. Internet: http://www.apta.org

Chapter 8

PHYSICIAN ASSISTANTS

SIGNIFICANT POINTS

- The typical physician assistant program lasts about 2 years and usually requires at least 2 years of college and some healthcare experience for admission.
- Earnings are high and job opportunities should be good.

NATURE OF THE WORK

Physician assistants (PAs) provide healthcare services under the supervision of physicians. They should not be confused with medical assistants, who perform routine clinical and clerical tasks. PAs are formally trained to provide diagnostic, therapeutic, and preventive healthcare services, as delegated by a physician. Working as members of the healthcare team, they take medical histories, examine and treat patients, order and interpret laboratory tests and x rays, make diagnoses, and prescribe medications. They also treat minor injuries by suturing, splinting, and casting. PAs record progress notes, instruct and counsel patients, and order or carry out therapy. In 47 States and the District of Columbia, physician assistants may prescribe medications. PAs also may have managerial duties. Some order medical and laboratory supplies and equipment and may supervise technicians and assistants. Physician assistants work under the supervision of a physician. However, PAs may be the principal care providers in rural or inner city clinics, where a physician is present for only 1 or 2 days each week. In such cases, the PA confers with the supervising physician and other medical professionals as needed or as required by law. PAs also may make house calls or go to hospitals and nursing homes to check on patients and report back to the physician. The duties of physician assistants are determined by the supervising physician and by State law. Aspiring PAs should investigate the laws and regulations in the States in which they wish to practice. Many PAs work in primary care areas such as general internal medicine, pediatrics, and family medicine. Others work in specialty areas, such as general and thoracic surgery, emergency medicine, orthopedics, and geriatrics. PAs specializing in surgery provide pre- and postoperative care, and may work as first or second assistants during major surgery.

WORKING CONDITIONS

Although PAs usually work in a comfortable, well-lighted environment, those in surgery often stand for long periods, and others do considerable walking. Schedules vary according to practice setting, and often depend on the hours of the supervising physician. The workweek of PAs in physicians' offices may include weekends, night hours, or early morning hospital rounds to visit patients. These workers also may be on call. PAs in clinics usually work a 40-hour week.

EMPLOYMENT

Physician assistants held about 58,000 jobs in 2000. The number of jobs is greater than the number of practicing PAs because some hold two or more jobs. For example, some PAs work with a supervising physician, but also work in another practice, clinic, or hospital. According to the American Academy of Physician Assistants, there were about 40,469 certified PAs in clinical practice as of January 2000. Almost 56 percent of jobs for PA's were in the offices and clinics of physicians, dentists, or other health practitioners. About 32 percent were in hospitals. The rest were mostly in public health clinics, temporary help agencies, schools, prisons, home healthcare agencies, and the U.S. Department of Veterans Affairs. According to the American Academy of Physician Assistants, about one-third of all PAs provide healthcare to communities with fewer than 50,000 residents, in which physicians may be in limited supply.

TRAINING, OTHER QUALIFICATIONS AND ADVANCEMENT

All States require that new PAs complete an accredited, formal education program. As of July 2001, there were 129 accredited or provisionally accredited educational programs for physician assistants; 64 of these programs offered a master's degree. The rest offered either a bachelor's degree or an associate degree. Most PA graduates have at least a bachelor's degree. Admission requirements vary, but many programs require 2 years of college and some work experience in the healthcare field. Students should take courses in biology, English, chemistry, math, psychology, and social sciences. More than two-thirds of all applicants hold a bachelor's or master's degree. Many applicants are former emergency medical technicians, other allied health professionals, or nurses.

PA programs usually last at least 2 years. Most programs are in schools of allied health, academic health centers, medical schools, or 4-year colleges; a few are in community colleges, the military, or hospitals. Many accredited PA programs have clinical teaching affiliations with medical schools. PA education includes classroom instruction in biochemistry, pathology, human anatomy, physiology, microbiology, clinical pharmacology, clinical medicine, geriatric and home healthcare, disease prevention, and medical ethics. Students obtain supervised clinical training in several areas, including primary care medicine, inpatient medicine, surgery, obstetrics and gynecology, geriatrics, emergency medicine, psychiatry, and pediatrics. Sometimes, PA students serve one or more of these "rotations" under the supervision of a physician who is seeking to hire a PA. These rotations often lead to permanent employment. All States and the District of Columbia have legislation governing the qualifications or practice of physician assistants. All jurisdictions require physician assistants to pass the Physician Assistants National Certifying Examination, administered by the National Commission on Certification of Physician Assistants (NCCPA)- open to graduates of accredited PA educational programs. Only those successfully completing the examination may use the credential "Physician Assistant-Certified (PA-C)."

In order to remain certified, PAs must complete 100 hours of continuing medical education every 2 years. Every 6 years, they must pass a recertification examination or complete an alternate program combining learning experiences and a take-home examination.

Some PA's pursue additional education in a specialty area such as surgery, neonatology, or emergency medicine. PA postgraduate residency training programs are available in areas such as internal medicine, rural primary care, emergency medicine, surgery, pediatrics, neonatology, and occupational medicine. Candidates must be graduates of an accredited program and be certified by the NCCPA.

Physician assistants need leadership skills, self-confidence, and emotional stability. They must be willing to continue studying throughout their career to keep up with medical advances. As they attain greater clinical knowledge and experience, PAs can advance to added responsibilities and higher earnings. However, by the very nature of the profession, clinically practicing PAs always are supervised by physicians.

JOB OUTLOOK

Employment opportunities are expected to be good for physician assistants, particularly in areas or settings that have difficulty attracting physicians, such as rural and inner city clinics. Employment of PAs is expected to grow much faster than the average for all occupations through the year 2010 due to anticipated expansion of the health services industry and an emphasis on cost containment. Physicians and institutions are expected to employ more PAs to provide primary care and to assist with medical and surgical procedures because PAs are cost-effective and productive members of the healthcare team. Physician assistants can relieve physicians of routine duties and procedures. Telemedicine-using technology to facilitate interactive consultations between physicians and physician assistants-also will expand the use of physician assistants. Besides the traditional office-based setting, PAs should find a growing number of jobs in institutional settings such as hospitals, academic medical centers, public clinics, and prisons. Additional PAs may be needed to augment medical staffing in inpatient teaching hospital settings if the number of physician residents is reduced. In addition, State-imposed legal limitations on the numbers of hours worked by physician residents are increasingly common and encourage hospitals to use PAs to supply some physician resident services. Opportunities will be best in States that allow PAs a wider scope of practice.

EARNINGS

Median annual earnings of physician assistants were $61,910 in 2000. The middle 50 percent earned between $47,970 and $73,890. The lowest 10 percent earned less than $32,690, and the highest 10 percent earned more than $88,100. Median annual earnings of physician assistants in 2000 were $64,430 in offices and clinics of medical doctors and $61,460 in hospitals. According to the American Academy of Physician Assistants, median income for physician assistants in full- time clinical practice in 2000 was about $65,177; median income for first-year graduates was about $56,977. Income varies by specialty, practice setting, geographical location, and years of experience.

RELATED OCCUPATIONS

Other health workers who provide direct patient care that requires a similar level of skill and training include occupational therapists, physical therapists, and speech- language pathologists and audiologists.

SOURCES OF ADDITIONAL INFORMATION

For information on a career as a physician assistant, contact: American Academy of Physician Assistants Information Center, 950 North Washington St., Alexandria, VA 22314-1552. Internet: http://www.aapa.org

For a list of accredited programs and a catalog of individual PA training programs, contact: Association of Physician Assistant Programs, 950 North Washington St., Alexandria, VA 22314-1552. Internet: http://www.apap.org

For eligibility requirements and a description of the Physician Assistant National Certifying Examination, contact: National Commission on Certification of Physician Assistants, Inc., 157 Technology Pkwy., Suite 800, Norcross, GA 30092-2913. Internet: http://www.nccpa.net

Chapter 9

PHYSICIANS AND SURGEONS

SIGNIFICANT POINTS

- Physicians are much more likely to work as salaried employees of group medical practices, clinics, or integrated healthcare systems than in the past.
- Formal education and training requirements are among the most demanding of any occupation, but earnings are among the highest.

NATURE OF THE WORK

Physicians and surgeons serve a fundamental role in our society and have an effect upon all our lives. They diagnose illnesses and prescribe and administer treatment for people suffering from injury or disease. Physicians examine patients, obtain medical histories, and order, perform, and interpret diagnostic tests. They counsel patients on diet, hygiene, and preventive healthcare.

There are two types of physicians: The M.D.-Doctor of Medicine-and the D.O.-Doctor of Osteopathic Medicine. M.D.s also are known as allopathic physicians. While both M.D.s and D.O.s may use all accepted methods of treatment, including drugs and surgery, D.O.s place special emphasis on the body's musculoskeletal system, preventive medicine, and holistic patient care.

Table 1. Percent distribution of M.D.s by specialty, 1999, Percent Total 100.0

Primary care		
	Internal medicine	16.1
	General and family practice	10.7
	Pediatrics	7.5
Medical specialties		
	Allergy	0.5
	Cardiovascular diseases	2.5
	Dermatology	1.2
	Gastroenterology	1.3
	Obstetrics and gynecology	4.9
	Pediatric cardiology	0.2
	Pulmonary diseases	1.0
Surgical specialties		
	Colon and rectal surgery	0.1
	General surgery	4.9
	Neurological surgery	0.6
	Ophthalmology	2.2
	Orthopedic surgery	2.7
	Otolaryngology	1.1
	Plastic surgery	0.7
	Thoracic surgery	0.1
	Urological surgery	1.3
Other specialties		
	Aerospace medicine	0.1
	Anesthesiology	4.4
	Child psychiatry	0.7
	Diagnostic radiology	2.6
	Emergency medicine	2.8
	Forensic pathology	0.1
	General preventive medicine	0.4
	Neurology	1.5
	Nuclear medicine	0.2
	Occupational medicine	0.4
	Pathology	2.3
	Physical medicine and rehabilitation	0.8
	Psychiatry	4.9
	Public health	0.2
	Radiology	1.0
	Radiation oncology	0.5
	Other specialty	0.7
	Unspecified/unknown/inactive	16.0

Source: American Medical Association

About a third of M.D.s-and more than half of D.O.s-are primary care physicians. They practice general and family medicine, general internal medicine, or general pediatrics and usually are the first health professionals patients consult. Primary care physicians tend to see the same patients on a regular basis for preventive care and to treat a variety of ailments. General and family practitioners emphasize comprehensive healthcare for patients of all ages and for the family as a group. Those in general internal medicine provide care mainly for adults who may have problems associated with the body's organs. General pediatricians focus on the whole range of children's health issues. When appropriate, primary care physicians refer patients to specialists, who are experts in medical fields such as obstetrics and gynecology, cardiology, psychiatry, or surgery (table 1).

D.O.s are more likely to be primary care providers than M.D.s, although they can be found in all specialties. Over half of D.O.s practice general or family medicine, general internal medicine, or general pediatrics. Common specialties for D.O.s include emergency medicine, anesthesiology, obstetrics and gynecology, psychiatry, and surgery.

Surgeons are physicians who specialize in the treatment of injury, disease, and deformity through operations. With patients under general or local anesthesia, a surgeon operates using a variety of instruments to correct physical deformities, repair bone and tissue after injuries, or perform preventive surgeries on patients with debilitating diseases or disorders. Though a large number perform general surgery, many surgeons choose to specialize in a specific area. One of the most prevalent specialties is orthopedic surgery, the treatment of the skeletal system and associated organs. Others include ophthalmology (treatment of the eye), neurological surgery (treatment of the brain and nervous system), and plastic or reconstructive surgery. Surgeons, like primary care and other specialist physicians, also examine patients, perform, and interpret diagnostic tests, and counsel patients on preventive healthcare.

WORKING CONDITIONS

Many physicians work in small private offices or clinics, often assisted by a small staff of nurses and other administrative personnel. Increasingly, physicians practice in groups or healthcare organizations that provide back-up coverage and allow for more time off. These physicians often work as part of a team coordinating care for a population of patients; they are less independent than solo practitioners of the past.

Surgeons typically work in well-lighted, sterile environments while performing surgery and often stand for long periods. Most work in hospitals or in surgical outpatient centers. Many physicians and surgeons work long, irregular hours. Almost one-third of physicians worked 60 hours or more a week in 2000. They must travel frequently between office and hospital to care for their patients. Physicians and surgeons who are on call deal with many patients' concerns over the phone, and may make emergency visits to hospitals or nursing homes.

EMPLOYMENT

Physicians and surgeons held about 598,000 jobs in 2000. About 7 out of 10 were in office-based practice and about 2 out of 10 were employed by hospitals. Others practiced in the Federal Government, most in U.S. Department of Veterans Affairs hospitals and clinics or in the Public Health Service of the Department of Health and Human Services.

A growing number of physicians are partners or salaried employees of group practices. Organized as clinics or as groups of physicians, medical groups can afford expensive medical equipment and realize other business advantages. Also, hospitals are integrating physician practices into healthcare networks that provide a continuum of care both inside and outside the hospital setting.

The New England and Middle Atlantic States have the highest ratio of physicians to population; the South Central States have the lowest. D.O.s are more likely than M.D.s to practice in small cities and towns and in rural areas. M.D.s tend to locate in urban areas, close to hospital and educational centers.

TRAINING AND OTHER QUALIFICATIONS

It takes many years of education and training to become a physician: 4 years of undergraduate school, 4 years of medical school, and 3 to 8 years of internship and residency, depending on the specialty selected. A few medical schools offer a combined undergraduate and medical school program that lasts 6 years instead of the customary 8 years.

Premedical students must complete undergraduate work in physics, biology, mathematics, English, and inorganic and organic chemistry. Students also take courses in the humanities and the social sciences. Some students also volunteer at local hospitals or clinics to gain practical experience in the health professions.

The minimum educational requirement for entry into a medical school is 3 years of college; most applicants, however, have at least a bachelor's degree, and many have advanced degrees. There are 144 medical schools in the United States-125 teach allopathic medicine and award a Doctor of Medicine (M.D.) degree; 19 teach osteopathic medicine and award the Doctor of Osteopathic Medicine (D.O.) degree. Acceptance to medical school is very competitive. Applicants must submit transcripts, scores from the Medical College Admission Test, and letters of recommendation. Schools also consider character, personality, leadership qualities, and participation in extracurricular activities. Most schools require an interview with members of the admissions committee.

Students spend most of the first 2 years of medical school in laboratories and classrooms taking courses such as anatomy, biochemistry, physiology, pharmacology, psychology, microbiology, pathology, medical ethics, and laws governing medicine. They also learn to take medical histories, examine patients, and diagnose illness. During the last 2 years, students work with patients under the supervision of experienced physicians in hospitals and clinics to learn acute, chronic, preventive, and rehabilitative care. Through rotations in internal medicine, family practice, obstetrics and gynecology, pediatrics, psychiatry, and surgery, they gain experience in the diagnosis and treatment of illness.

Following medical school, almost all M.D.s enter a residency-graduate medical education in a specialty that takes the form of paid on-the-job training, usually in a hospital. Most D.O.s serve a 12-month rotating internship after graduation before entering a residency that may last 2 to 6 years. Physicians may benefit from residencies in managed care settings by gaining experience with this increasingly common type of medical practice.

All States, the District of Columbia, and U.S. territories license physicians. To be licensed, physicians must graduate from an accredited medical school, pass a licensing examination, and complete 1 to 7 years of graduate medical education. Although physicians licensed in one State can usually get a license to practice in another without further examination, some States limit reciprocity. Graduates of foreign medical schools usually can qualify for licensure after passing an examination and completing a U.S. residency.

M.D.s and D.O.s seeking board certification in a specialty may spend up to 7 years-depending on the specialty-in residency training. A final examination immediately after residency, or after 1 or 2 years of practice, also is necessary for board certification by the American Board of Medical Specialists (ABMS) or the - American Osteopathic Association (AOA). There are 24 specialty boards, ranging from allergy and immunology to urology. For certification in a subspecialty, physicians usually need another 1 to 2 years of residency.

A physician's training is costly and, whereas education costs have increased, student financial assistance has not. More than 80 percent of medical students borrow money to cover their expenses.

People who wish to become physicians must have a desire to serve patients, be self-motivated, and be able to survive the pressures and long hours of medical education and practice. Physicians also must have a good bedside manner, emotional stability, and the ability to make decisions in emergencies. Prospective physicians must be willing to study throughout their career to keep up with medical advances. They also will need to be flexible to respond to the changing demands of a rapidly evolving health care environment.

JOB OUTLOOK

Employment of physicians and surgeons will grow about as fast as the average for all occupations through the year 2010 due to continued expansion of the health care industries. The growing and aging population will drive overall growth in the demand for physician services. In addition, new technologies will permit more intensive care: Physicians will be able to do more tests, perform more procedures, and treat conditions previously regarded as untreatable. Although job prospects may be better for primary care physicians such as general and family practitioners, general pediatricians, and general internists, a substantial number of jobs for specialists will also be created in response to patient demand for access to specialty care.

The number of physicians in training has leveled off and is likely to decrease over the next few years, alleviating the effects of any physician oversupply. However, future physicians may be more likely to work fewer hours, retire earlier, have lower earnings, or have to practice in underserved areas. Opportunities should be good in rural and low income areas, because some physicians find these areas unattractive due to lower earnings potential, isolation from medical colleagues, or other reasons.

Unlike their predecessors, newly trained physicians face radically different choices of where and how to practice. New physicians are much less likely to enter solo practice and more likely to take salaried jobs in group medical practices, clinics, and integrated healthcare systems.

EARNINGS

Physicians have among the highest earnings of any occupation. According to the latest data available from the American Medical Association, median income, after expenses, for allopathic physicians was about $160,000 in 1998. The middle 50 percent earned between $120,000 and $240,000 a year. Self-employed physicians-those who own or are part owners of their medical practice-had higher median incomes than salaried physicians. Earnings vary according to number of years in practice, geographic region, hours worked, and skill, personality, and professional reputation. As shown in table 2, median income of allopathic physicians, after expenses, also varies by specialty.

Table 2. Median net income of M.D.s after expenses, 1998

All physicians	$160,000
Surgery	$240,000
Radiology	$230,000
Anesthesiology	$210,000
Obstetrics/gynecology	$200,000
Emergency medicine	$184,000
Pathology	$184,000
General internal medicine	$140,000
General/Family practice	$130,000
Psychiatry	$130,000
Pediatrics	$126,000

Source: American Medical Association

RELATED OCCUPATIONS

Physicians work to prevent, diagnose, and treat diseases, disorders, and injuries. Professionals in other occupations requiring similar skills and critical judgment include chiropractors, dentists, optometrists, physician assistants, podiatrists, speech-language pathologists and audiologists, and veterinarians.

SOURCES OF ADDITIONAL INFORMATION

For a list of medical schools and residency programs, as well as general information on premedical education, financial aid, and medicine as a career, contact:

- Association of American Medical Colleges, Section for Student Services, 2450 N St. NW., Washington, DC 20037-1126. Internet: http://www.aamc.org
- American Association of Colleges of Osteopathic Medicine, 5550 Friendship Blvd., Suite 310, Chevy Chase, MD 20815-7321. Internet: http://www.aacom.org

For general information on physicians, contact:

- American Medical Association, Department of Communications and Public Relations, 515 N. State St., Chicago, IL 60610. Internet: http://www.ama-assn.org
- American Osteopathic Association, Department of Public Relations, 142 East Ontario St., Chicago, IL 60611. Internet: http://www.aoa-net.org

Information on Federal scholarships and loans is available from the directors of student financial aid at schools of medicine. Information on licensing is available from State boards of examiners.

Chapter 10

PODIATRISTS

SIGNIFICANT POINTS

- A limited number of job openings for podiatrists is expected because the occupation is small and most podiatrists remain in the occupation until they retire.
- Most podiatrists are solo practitioners, although more are entering partnerships and multispecialty group practices.
- Podiatrists enjoy very high earnings.

NATURE OF THE WORK

Americans spend a great deal of time on their feet. As the Nation becomes more active across all age groups, the need for footcare will become increasingly important to maintaining a healthy lifestyle.

The human foot is a complex structure. It contains 26 bones-plus muscles, nerves, ligaments, and blood vessels-and is designed for balance and mobility. The 52 bones in your feet make up about one-fourth of all the bones in your body. Podiatrists, also known as doctors of podiatric medicine (DPMs), diagnose and treat disorders, diseases, and injuries of the foot and lower leg to keep this part of the body working properly.

Podiatrists treat corns, calluses, ingrown toenails, bunions, heel spurs, and arch problems; ankle and foot injuries, deformities and infections; and foot complaints associated with diseases such as diabetes. To treat these problems, podiatrists prescribe drugs, order physical therapy, set fractures, and perform surgery. They also fit corrective inserts called orthotics, design plaster casts and strappings to correct deformities, and design custom-made shoes. Podiatrists may use a force plate to help design the orthotics. Patients walk across a plate connected to a computer that "reads" the patients' feet, picking up pressure points and weight distribution. From the computer readout, podiatrists order the correct design or recommend treatment.

To diagnose a foot problem, podiatrists also order x rays and laboratory tests. The foot may be the first area to show signs of serious conditions such as arthritis, diabetes, and heart disease. For example, diabetics are prone to foot ulcers and infections due to poor circulation. Podiatrists consult with and refer patients to other health practitioners when they detect symptoms of these disorders.

Most podiatrists have a solo practice, although more are forming group practices with other podiatrists or health practitioners. Some specialize in surgery, orthopedics, primary care, or public health. Besides these board-certified specialties, podiatrists may practice a subspecialty such as sports medicine, pediatrics, dermatology, radiology, geriatrics, or diabetic foot care.

Podiatrists who are in private practice are responsible for running a small business. They may hire employees, order supplies, and keep records, among other tasks. In addition, some educate the community on the benefits of footcare through speaking engagements and advertising.

WORKING CONDITIONS

Podiatrists usually work in their own offices. They also may spend time visiting patients in nursing homes or performing surgery at a hospital, but usually have fewer after-hours emergencies than other doctors. Those with private practices set their own hours, but may work evenings and weekends to meet the needs of their patients.

EMPLOYMENT

Podiatrists held about 18,000 jobs in 2000. Most podiatrists are solo practitioners, although more are entering partnerships and multispecialty group practices. Others are employed in hospitals, nursing homes, the U.S. Public Health Service, and the U.S. Department of Veterans Affairs.

TRAINING, OTHER QUALIFICATIONS AND ADVANCEMENT

All States and the District of Columbia require a license for the practice of podiatric medicine. Each defines its own licensing requirements. Generally, the applicant must be a graduate of an accredited college of podiatric medicine and pass written and oral examinations. Some States permit applicants to substitute the examination of the National Board of Podiatric Examiners, given in the second and fourth years of podiatric medical college, for part or all of the written State examination. Most States also require completion of a postdoctoral residency program. Many States grant reciprocity to podiatrists who are licensed in another State. Most States require continuing education for licensure renewal.

Prerequisites for admission to a college of podiatric medicine include the completion of at least 90 semester hours of undergraduate study, an acceptable grade point average, and suitable scores on the Medical College Admission Test (MCAT). All require 8 semester hours each of biology, inorganic chemistry, organic chemistry, and physics, and 6 hours of English. The science courses should be those designed for premedical students. Potential podiatric medical students may also be evaluated on the basis of extracurricular and community activities, personal interviews, and letters of recommendation. More than 90 percent of podiatric students have at least a bachelor's degree.

Colleges of podiatric medicine offer a 4-year program whose core curriculum is similar to that in other schools of medicine. During the first 2 years, students receive classroom instruction in basic sciences, including anatomy, chemistry, pathology, and pharmacology. Third- and fourth-year students have clinical rotations in private practices, hospitals, and clinics. During these rotations, they learn how to take general and podiatric histories, perform routine physical examinations, interpret tests and findings, make diagnoses, and perform therapeutic procedures. Graduates receive the doctor of podiatric medicine (DPM) degree.

Most graduates complete a hospital residency program after receiving a DPM. Residency programs last from 1 to 3 years. Residents receive advanced training in podiatric medicine and surgery and serve clinical rotations in anesthesiology, internal medicine, pathology, radiology, emergency medicine, and orthopedic and general surgery. Residencies lasting more than 1 year provide more extensive training in specialty areas.

There are a number of certifying boards for the podiatric specialties of orthopedics, primary medicine, or surgery. Certification means that the DPM meets higher standards than those required for licensure. Each board requires advanced training, completion of written and oral examinations, and experience as a practicing podiatrist. Most managed care organizations prefer board-certified podiatrists. People planning a career in podiatry should have scientific aptitude, manual dexterity, interpersonal skills, and good business sense.

Podiatrists may advance to become professors at colleges of podiatric medicine, department chiefs of hospitals, or general health administrators.

JOB OUTLOOK

Employment of podiatrists is expected to grow about as fast as the average for all occupations through 2010. More people will turn to podiatrists for footcare as the elderly population grows. The elderly have more years of wear and tear on their feet and legs than most younger people, so they are more prone to foot ailments. Injuries sustained by an increasing number of men and women of all ages leading active lifestyles will also spur demand for podiatric care.

Medicare and most private health insurance programs cover acute medical and surgical foot services, as well as diagnostic x rays and leg braces. Details of such coverage vary among plans. However, routine foot care-including the removal of corns and calluses-is ordinarily not covered, unless the patient has a systemic condition that has resulted in severe circulatory problems or areas of desensitization in the legs or feet. Like dental services, podiatric care is more dependent on disposable income than other medical services.

Employment of podiatrists would grow even faster were it not for continued emphasis on controlling the costs of specialty healthcare. Insurers will balance the cost of sending patients to podiatrists against the cost and availability of substitute practitioners, such as physicians and physical therapists. Opportunities will be better for board-certified podiatrists, because many managed care organizations require board-certification. Opportunities for newly trained podiatrists will be better in group medical practices, clinics, and health networks than in a traditional solo practice. Establishing a practice will be most difficult in the areas surrounding colleges of podiatric medicine because podiatrists are concentrated in these locations.

Over the next 10 years, members of the "baby boom" generation will begin to retire, creating vacancies. Relatively few job openings from this source are expected, however, because the occupation is small.

EARNINGS

Median annual earnings of salaried podiatrists were $107,560 in 2000. The middle 50 percent earned between $77,440 and $134,900 a year. According to a survey by Podiatry Management magazine, median net income of podiatrists in solo practice, including the self-employed, was $89,681 in 2000. Those in group practices or partnerships earned median net income of $96,200 in 2000. Self-employed podiatrists must provide for their own health insurance and retirement.

RELATED OCCUPATIONS

Workers in other occupations who apply scientific knowledge to prevent, diagnose, and treat disorders and injuries are chiropractors, dentists, optometrists, physicians and surgeons, and veterinarians.

SOURCES OF ADDITIONAL INFORMATION

For information on podiatric medicine as a career, contact: American Podiatric Medical Association, 9312 Old Georgetown Rd., Bethesda, MD 20814-1621. Internet: http://www.apma.org

Information on colleges of podiatric medicine, entrance requirements, curriculums, and student financial aid is available from: American Association of Colleges of Podiatric Medicine, 1350 Piccard Dr., Suite 322, Rockville, MD 20850-4307. Internet: http://www.aacpm.org

Chapter 11

RECREATIONAL THERAPISTS

SIGNIFICANT POINTS

- Employment growth is expected in assisted living, physical and psychiatric rehabilitation, and services for people with disabilities.
- Opportunities should be best for persons with a bachelor's degree in therapeutic recreation or in recreation with a concentration in therapeutic recreation.

NATURE OF THE WORK

Recreational therapists, also referred to as therapeutic recreation specialists, provide treatment services and recreation activities to individuals with disabilities, illnesses, or other disabling conditions. Therapists treat and maintain the physical, mental, and emotional well-being of clients using a variety of techniques, including the use of arts and crafts, animals, sports, games, dance and movement, drama, music, and community outings. Therapists help individuals reduce depression, stress, and anxiety. They also help individuals recover basic motor functioning and reasoning abilities, build confidence, and socialize effectively to enable greater independence, as well as to reduce or eliminate the effects of illness or disability. Additionally, they help integrate people with disabilities into the community by helping them use community resources and recreational activities. Recreational therapists should not be confused with recreation and fitness workers, who organize recreational activities primarily for enjoyment.

In acute healthcare settings, such as hospitals and rehabilitation centers, recreational therapists treat and rehabilitate individuals with specific health conditions, usually in conjunction or collaboration with physicians, nurses, psychologists, social workers, and physical and occupational therapists. In long-term and residential care facilities, recreational therapists use leisure activities-especially structured group programs-to improve and maintain general health and well-being. They may also treat clients and provide interventions to prevent further medical problems and secondary complications related to illness and disabilities.

Recreational therapists assess clients, based on information from standardized assessments, observations, medical records, medical staff, family, and clients themselves. They then develop and carry out therapeutic interventions consistent with client needs and interests. For example, clients isolated from others, or with limited social skills, may be encouraged to play games with others, or right-handed persons with right-side paralysis may be instructed to adapt to using their nonaffected left side to throw a ball or swing a racket. Recreational therapists may instruct patients in relaxation techniques to reduce stress and tension, stretching and limbering exercises, proper body mechanics for participation in recreation activities, pacing and energy conservation techniques, and individual as well as team activities. Additionally, therapists observe and document patients' participation, reactions, and progress.

Community-based therapeutic recreation specialists may work in park and recreation departments, special education programs for school districts, or programs for older adults and people with disabilities. Included in the latter group are programs and facilities such as assisted living, adult day care, and substance abuse rehabilitation centers. In these programs, therapists use interventions to develop specific skills while providing opportunities for exercise, mental stimulation, creativity, and fun. Although most therapists are employed in other areas, those who work in schools help counselors, teachers, and parents address the special needs of students-most importantly, easing the transition into adult life for disabled students.

WORKING CONDITIONS

Recreational therapists provide services in special activity rooms but also plan activities and prepare documentation in offices. When working with clients during community integration programs, they may travel locally to instruct clients on the accessibility of public transportation and other public areas, such as parks, playgrounds, swimming pools, restaurants, and theaters.

Therapists often lift and carry equipment as well as lead recreational activities. Recreational therapists generally work a 40-hour week that may include some evenings, weekends, and holidays.

EMPLOYMENT

Recreational therapists held about 29,000 jobs in 2000. Almost 40 percent of salaried jobs for therapists were in nursing and personal care facilities, and over 30 percent were in hospitals. Others worked in residential facilities, community mental health centers, adult daycare programs, correctional facilities, community programs for people with disabilities, and substance abuse centers. Only a small number of therapists were self-employed, generally contracting with long-term care facilities or community agencies to develop and oversee programs.

TRAINING, OTHER QUALIFICATIONS AND ADVANCEMENT

A bachelor's degree in therapeutic recreation, or in recreation with a concentration in therapeutic recreation, is the usual requirement for entry-level positions. Persons may qualify for paraprofessional positions with an associate degree in therapeutic recreation or a health care related field. An associate degree in recreational therapy; training in art, drama, or music therapy; or qualifying work experience may be sufficient for activity director positions in nursing homes.

There are approximately 160 programs that prepare recreational therapists. Most offer bachelor's degrees, although some also offer associate, master's, or doctoral degrees. Programs include courses in assessment, treatment and program planning, intervention design, and evaluation. Students also study human anatomy, physiology, abnormal psychology, medical and psychiatric terminology, characteristics of illnesses and disabilities, professional ethics, and the use of assistive devices and technology.

Most employers prefer to hire candidates who are certified therapeutic recreation specialists (CTRS). The National Council for Therapeutic

Recreation Certification (NCTRC) certifies therapeutic recreation specialists. To presently become certified, specialists must have a bachelor's degree, pass a written certification examination, and complete an internship of at least 360 hours. Beginning in 2003, however, specialists will be required to complete an internship of at least 480 hours, in addition to the degree and examination requirements.

Recreational therapists should be comfortable working with persons who are ill or have disabilities. Therapists must be patient, tactful, and persuasive when working with people who have a variety of special needs. Ingenuity, a sense of humor, and imagination are needed to adapt activities to individual needs; and good physical coordination is necessary to demonstrate or participate in recreational activities. Therapists may advance to supervisory or administrative positions. Some teach, conduct research, or consult for health or social service agencies.

JOB OUTLOOK

Overall employment of recreational therapists is expected to grow more slowly than the average for all occupations through the year 2010. Employment will decline slightly in the two largest sectors employing recreational therapists, hospitals and nursing homes, as services shift to outpatient settings and employers emphasize cost containment. However, fast employment growth is expected in assisted living, outpatient physical and psychiatric rehabilitation, and services for people with disabilities. Opportunities should be best for persons with a bachelor's degree in therapeutic recreation or in recreation with an option in therapeutic recreation. Healthcare facilities will provide a growing number of jobs in hospital-based adult day care and outpatient programs and in units offering short-term mental health and alcohol or drug abuse services. Rehabilitation, home healthcare, transitional programs, and psychiatric facilities will provide additional jobs.

The rapidly growing number of older adults is expected to spur job growth for therapeutic recreation specialists and recreational therapy paraprofessionals in assisted living facilities, adult daycare programs, and social service agencies. Continued growth also is expected in community residential facilities, as well as day care programs for individuals with disabilities.

EARNINGS

Median annual earnings of recreational therapists were $28,650 in 2000. The middle 50 percent earned between $21,780 and $36,070 a year. The lowest 10 percent earned less than $17,010, and the highest 10 percent earned more than $43,810 a year. Median annual earnings for recreational therapists in 2000 were $32,520 in hospitals and $23,240 in nursing and personal care facilities.

RELATED OCCUPATIONS

Recreational therapists primarily design activities to help people with disabilities lead more fulfilling and independent lives. Other workers who have similar jobs are occupational therapists, physical therapists, recreation and fitness workers, and rehabilitation counselors.

SOURCES OF ADDITIONAL INFORMATION

For information on how to order materials describing careers and academic programs in recreational therapy, write to:

- American Therapeutic Recreation Association, 1414 Prince St., Suite 204, Alexandria, VA 22314-2853. Internet: http://www.atra-tr.org
- National Therapeutic Recreation Society, 22377 Belmont Ridge Rd., Ashburn, VA 20148-4501. Internet: http://www.nrpa.org/index.cfm?publicationid=21

Certification information may be obtained from: National Council for Therapeutic Recreation Certification, 7 Elmwood Dr., New City, NY 10956. Internet: http://www.nctrc.org

Chapter 12

REGISTERED NURSES

SIGNIFICANT POINTS

- The largest health care occupation, with more than 2 million jobs.
- One of the 10 occupations projected to have the largest numbers of new jobs.
- Job opportunities are expected to be very good.
- Earnings are above average, particularly for advanced practice nurses, who have additional education or training.

NATURE OF THE WORK

Registered nurses (RNs) work to promote health, prevent disease, and help patients cope with illness. They are advocates and health educators for patients, families, and communities. When providing direct patient care, they observe, assess, and record symptoms, reactions, and progress; assist physicians during treatments and examinations; administer medications; and assist in convalescence and rehabilitation. RNs also develop and manage nursing care plans; instruct patients and their families in proper care; and help individuals and groups take steps to improve or maintain their health.

While State laws govern the tasks that RNs may perform, it is usually the work setting that determines their daily job duties. Hospital nurses form the largest group of nurses. Most are staff nurses, who provide bedside nursing care and carry out medical regimens. They also may supervise licensed practical nurses and nursing aides. Hospital nurses usually are assigned to one area, such as surgery, maternity, pediatrics, emergency room, intensive care, or treatment of cancer patients. Some may rotate among departments.

Office nurses care for outpatients in physicians' offices, clinics, surgicenters, and emergency medical centers. They prepare patients for and assist with examinations, administer injections and medications, dress wounds and incisions, assist with minor surgery, and maintain records. Some also perform routine laboratory and office work.

Nursing home nurses manage nursing care for residents with conditions ranging from a fracture to Alzheimer's disease. Although they often spend much of their time on administrative and supervisory tasks, RNs also assess residents' health condition, develop treatment plans, supervise licensed practical nurses and nursing aides, and perform difficult procedures such as starting intravenous fluids.

They also work in specialty- care departments, such as long-term rehabilitation units for patients with strokes and head-injuries. Home health nurses provide periodic services to patients at home. After assessing patients' home environments, they care for and instruct patients and their families. Home health nurses care for a broad range of patients, such as those recovering from illnesses and accidents, cancer, and childbirth. They must be able to work independently, and may supervise home health aides.

Public health nurses work in government and private agencies and clinics, schools, retirement communities, and other community settings. They focus on populations, working with individuals, groups, and families to improve the overall health of communities. They also work as partners with communities to plan and implement programs. Public health nurses instruct individuals, families, and other groups regarding health issues, disease prevention, nutrition, and childcare. They arrange for immunizations, blood pressure testing, and other health screening. These nurses also work with community leaders, teachers, parents, and physicians in community health education.

Occupational health or industrial nurses provide nursing care at worksites to employees, customers, and others with minor injuries and illnesses. They provide emergency care, prepare accident reports, and arrange for further care if necessary. They also offer health counseling, assist with health examinations and inoculations, and assess work environments to identify potential health or safety problems.

Head nurses or nurse supervisors direct nursing activities. They plan work schedules and assign duties to nurses and aides, provide or arrange for training, and visit patients to observe nurses and to ensure the proper delivery of care. They also may see that records are maintained and equipment and supplies are ordered. At the advanced level, nurse practitioners provide basic primary healthcare. They diagnose and treat common acute illnesses and injuries. Nurse practitioners also can prescribe medications-but certification and licensing requirements vary by State. Other advanced practice nurses include clinical nurse specialists, certified registered nurse anesthetists, and certified nurse-midwives. Advanced practice nurses must meet higher educational and clinical practice requirements beyond the basic nursing education and licensing required of all RNs.

WORKING CONDITIONS

Most nurses work in well-lighted, comfortable healthcare facilities. Home health and public health nurses travel to patients' homes, schools, community centers, and other sites. Nurses may spend considerable time walking and standing. They need emotional stability to cope with human suffering, emergencies, and other stresses. Patients in hospitals and nursing homes require 24-hour care; consequently, nurses in these institutions may work nights, weekends, and holidays. RNs also may be on-call-available to work on short notice. Office, occupational health, and public health nurses are more likely to work regular business hours. Almost 1 in 10 RNs held more than one job in 2000. Nursing has its hazards, especially in hospitals, nursing homes, and clinics where nurses may care for individuals with infectious diseases. Nurses must observe rigid guidelines to guard against disease and other dangers, such as those posed by radiation, chemicals used for sterilization of instruments, and anesthetics. In addition, they are vulnerable to back injury when moving patients, shocks from electrical equipment, and hazards posed by compressed gases.

EMPLOYMENT

As the largest healthcare occupation, registered nurses held about 2.2 million jobs in 2000. About 3 out of 5 jobs were in hospitals, in inpatient and outpatient departments. Others were mostly in offices and clinics of physicians and other health practitioners, home healthcare agencies, nursing homes, temporary help agencies, schools, and government agencies. The remainder worked in residential care facilities, social service agencies, religious organizations, research facilities, management and public relations firms, insurance agencies, and private households. About 1 out of 4 RNs worked part time.

Training, Other Qualifications and Advancement

In all States and the District of Columbia, students must graduate from an approved nursing program and pass a national licensing examination to obtain a nursing license. Nurses may be licensed in more than one State, either by examination, by endorsement of a license issued by another State, or through a multi-State licensing agreement. All States require periodic license renewal, which may involve continuing education. There are three major educational paths to registered nursing: associate degree in nursing (A.D.N.), bachelor of science degree in nursing (B.S.N.), and diploma. A.D.N. programs, offered by community and junior colleges, take about 2 to 3 years. About half of the 1,700 RN programs in 2000 were at the A.D.N. level. B.S.N. programs, offered by colleges and universities, take 4 or 5 years. More than one-third of all programs in 2000 offered degrees at the bachelor's level. Diploma programs, administered in hospitals, last 2 to 3 years. Only a small number of programs offer diploma-level degrees. Generally, licensed graduates of any of the three program types qualify for entry-level positions as staff nurses. Many A.D.N. and diploma-educated nurses later enter bachelor's programs to prepare for a broader scope of nursing practice. They can often find a staff nurse position and then take advantage of tuition reimbursement programs to work toward a B.S.N. Individuals considering nursing should carefully weigh the pros and cons of enrolling in a B.S.N. program because, if they do so, their advancement opportunities usually are broader. In fact, some career paths are open only to nurses with bachelor's or advanced degrees. A bachelor's degree is often necessary for administrative positions, and it is a prerequisite for admission to graduate nursing programs in research, consulting, teaching, or a clinical specialization. Nursing education includes classroom instruction and supervised clinical experience in hospitals and other health facilities. Students take courses in anatomy, physiology, microbiology, chemistry, nutrition, psychology and other behavioral sciences, and nursing. Coursework also includes the liberal arts. Supervised clinical experience is provided in hospital departments such as pediatrics, psychiatry, maternity, and surgery. A growing number of programs include clinical experience in nursing homes, public health departments, home health agencies, and ambulatory clinics. Nurses should be caring and sympathetic. They must be able to accept responsibility, direct or supervise others, follow orders precisely, and determine when consultation is required. Experience and good performance can lead to promotion to more responsible positions. Nurses can advance, in management, to assistant head nurse or head nurse. From there, they can advance to assistant director, director, and vice president. Increasingly, management-level nursing positions require a graduate degree in nursing or health services administration. They also require leadership, negotiation skills, and good judgment. Graduate programs preparing executive-level nurses usually last 1 to 2 years. Within patient care, nurses can advance to clinical nurse specialist, nurse practitioner, certified nurse-midwife, or certified registered nurse anesthetist. These positions require 1 or 2 years of graduate education, leading to a master's degree or, in some instances, to a certificate. Some nurses move into the business side of healthcare. Their nursing expertise and experience on a healthcare team equip them to manage ambulatory, acute, home health, and chronic care services. Healthcare corporations employ nurses for health planning and development, marketing, and quality assurance. Other nurses work as college and university faculty or do research.

JOB OUTLOOK

Job opportunities for RNs are expected to be very good. Employment of registered nurses is expected to grow faster than the average for all occupations through 2010, and because the occupation is very large, many new jobs will result. Thousands of job openings also will result from the need to replace experienced nurses who leave the occupation, especially as the median age of the registered nurse population continues to rise. Some States report current and projected shortages of RNs, primarily due to an aging RN workforce and recent declines in nursing school enrollments. Imbalances between the supply of and demand for qualified workers should spur efforts to attract and retain qualified RNs. For example, employers may restructure workloads, improve compensation and working conditions, and subsidize training or continuing education. Faster than average growth will be driven by technological advances in patient care, which permit a greater number of medical problems to be treated, and an increasing emphasis on preventive care. In addition, the number of older people, who are much more likely than younger people to need nursing care, is projected to grow rapidly. Employment in hospitals, the largest sector, is expected to grow more slowly than in other healthcare sectors. While the intensity of nursing care is likely to increase, requiring more nurses per patient, the number of inpatients (those who remain in the hospital for more than 24 hours) is not likely to increase much. Patients are being discharged earlier and more procedures are being done on an outpatient basis, both in and outside hospitals. However, rapid growth is expected in hospital outpatient facilities, such as those providing same-day surgery, rehabilitation, and chemotherapy. Employment in home healthcare is expected to grow rapidly. This is in response to the growing number of older persons with functional disabilities, consumer preference for care in the home, and technological advances that make it possible to bring increasingly complex treatments into the home. The type of care demanded will require nurses who are able to perform complex procedures. Employment in nursing homes is expected to grow faster than average due to increases in the number of elderly, many of whom require long-term care. In addition, the financial pressure on hospitals to discharge patients as soon as possible should produce more nursing home admissions. Growth in units that provide specialized long-term rehabilitation for stroke and head injury patients or that treat Alzheimer's victims also will increase employment. An increasing proportion of sophisticated procedures, which once were performed only in hospitals, are being performed in physicians' offices and clinics, including ambulatory surgicenters and emergency medical centers. Accordingly, employment is expected to grow faster than average in these places as healthcare in general expands. In evolving integrated healthcare networks, nurses may rotate among employment settings. Because jobs in traditional hospital nursing positions are no longer the only option, RNs will need to be flexible. Opportunities should be excellent, particularly for nurses with advanced education and training.

EARNINGS

Median annual earnings of registered nurses were $44,840 in 2000. The middle 50 percent earned between $37,870 and $54,000. The lowest 10 percent earned less than $31,890, and the highest 10 percent earned more than $64,360. Median annual earnings in the industries employing the largest numbers of registered nurses in 2000 were as follows:

- Personnel supply services $46,860
- Hospitals $45,780
- Home health care services $43,640
- Offices and clinics of medical doctors $43,480
- Nursing and personal care facilities $41,330

Many employers offer flexible work schedules, childcare, educational benefits, and bonuses.

RELATED OCCUPATIONS

Workers in other healthcare occupations with responsibilities and duties related to those of registered nurses are emergency medical technicians and paramedics, occupational therapists, physical therapists, physician assistants, and respiratory therapists.

SOURCES OF ADDITIONAL INFORMATION

For information on a career as a registered nurse and nursing education, contact: National League for Nursing, 61 Broadway, New York, NY 10006. Internet: http://www.nln.org

For a list of B.S.N. and graduate nursing programs, write to: American Association of Colleges of Nursing, 1 Dupont Circle NW., Suite 530, Washington, DC 20036. Internet: http://www.aacn.nche.edu

Information on registered nurses also is available from: American Nurses Association, 600 Maryland Ave. SW., Washington, DC 20024-2571. Internet: http://www.nursingworld.org

Chapter 13

RESPIRATORY THERAPISTS

SIGNIFICANT POINTS

- Hospitals will continue to employ more than 8 out of 10 respiratory therapists, but a growing number of therapists will work in respiratory therapy clinics, nursing homes, home health agencies, and firms that supply respiratory equipment for home use.
- Job opportunities will be best for therapists with cardiopulmonary care skills or experience working with newborns and infants.

NATURE OF THE WORK

Respiratory therapists and respiratory therapy technicians-also known as respiratory care practitioners-evaluate, treat, and care for patients with breathing disorders. Respiratory therapists assume primary responsibility for all respiratory care treatments, including the supervision of respiratory therapy technicians. Respiratory therapy technicians provide specific, well-defined respiratory care procedures under the direction of respiratory therapists and physicians. In clinical practice, many of the daily duties of therapists and technicians overlap, although therapists generally have more experience than technicians. In this statement, the term respiratory therapists includes both respiratory therapists and respiratory therapy technicians.

To evaluate patients, respiratory therapists test the capacity of the lungs and analyze oxygen and carbon dioxide concentration. They also measure the patient's potential of hydrogen (pH), which indicates the acidity or alkalinity level of the blood. To measure lung capacity, patients breathe into an instrument that measures the volume and flow of oxygen during inhalation and exhalation. By comparing the reading with the norm for the patient's age, height, weight, and sex, respiratory therapists can determine whether lung deficiencies exist. To analyze oxygen, carbon dioxide, and pH levels, therapists draw an arterial blood sample, place it in a blood gas analyzer, and relay the results to a physician.

Respiratory therapists treat all types of patients, ranging from premature infants whose lungs are not fully developed, to elderly people whose lungs are diseased. These workers provide temporary relief to patients with chronic asthma or emphysema, as well as emergency care to patients who are victims of a heart attack, stroke, drowning, or shock.

To treat patients, respiratory therapists use oxygen or oxygen mixtures, chest physiotherapy, and aerosol medications. To increase a patient's concentration of oxygen, therapists place an oxygen mask or nasal cannula on a patient and set the oxygen flow at the level prescribed by a physician. Therapists also connect patients who cannot breathe on their own to ventilators that deliver pressurized oxygen into the lungs. They insert a tube into a patient's trachea, or windpipe; connect the tube to the ventilator; and set the rate, volume, and oxygen concentration of the oxygen mixture entering the patient's lungs.

Therapists regularly check on patients and equipment. If the patient appears to be having difficulty, or if the oxygen, carbon dioxide, or pH level of the blood is abnormal, they change the ventilator setting according to the doctor's order or check equipment for mechanical problems. In homecare, therapists teach patients and their families to use ventilators and other life support systems. Additionally, they visit several times a month to inspect and clean equipment and ensure its proper use and make emergency visits, if equipment problems arise.

Respiratory therapists perform chest physiotherapy on patients to remove mucus from their lungs and make it easier for them to breathe. For example, during surgery, anesthesia depresses respiration, so this treatment may be prescribed to help get the patient's lungs back to normal and to prevent congestion. Chest physiotherapy also helps patients suffering from lung diseases, such as cystic fibrosis, that cause mucus to collect in the lungs. In this procedure, therapists place patients in positions to help drain mucus, thump and vibrate patients' rib cages, and instruct them to cough. Respiratory therapists also administer aerosols-liquid medications suspended in a gas that forms a mist which is inhaled-and teach patients how to inhale the aerosol properly to assure its effectiveness.

In some hospitals, therapists perform tasks that fall outside their traditional role. Tasks are expanding into cardiopulmonary procedures like electrocardiograms and stress testing, as well as other tasks like drawing blood samples from patients. Therapists also keep records of materials used and charges to patients.

WORKING CONDITIONS

Respiratory therapists generally work between 35 and 40 hours a week. Because hospitals operate around the clock, therapists may work evenings, nights, or weekends. They spend long periods standing and walking between patients' rooms. In an emergency, therapists work under a great deal of stress.

Because gases used by respiratory therapists are stored under pressure, they are potentially hazardous. However, adherence to safety precautions and regular maintenance and testing of equipment minimize the risk of injury. As in many other health occupations, respiratory therapists run a risk of catching infectious diseases, but carefully following proper procedures minimizes this risk.

EMPLOYMENT

Respiratory therapists held about 110,000 jobs in 2000. More than 4 out of 5 jobs were in hospital departments of respiratory care, anesthesiology, or pulmonary medicine. Respiratory therapy clinics, offices of physicians, nursing homes, and firms that supply respiratory equipment for home use accounted for most of the remaining jobs.

TRAINING, OTHER QUALIFICATIONS AND ADVANCEMENT

Formal training is necessary for entry to this field. Training is offered at the postsecondary level by medical schools, colleges and universities, trade schools, vocational-technical institutes, and the Armed Forces. Formal training programs vary in length and in the credential or degree awarded.

Some programs award associate's or bachelor's degrees and prepare graduates for jobs as registered respiratory therapists (RRTs). Other, shorter programs award certificates and lead to jobs as entry-level certified respiratory therapists (CRTs). According to the Committee on Accreditation for Respiratory Care (CoARC), there were 334 accredited RRT programs and 102 accredited CRT programs in the United States in 2000.

Areas of study for respiratory therapy programs include human anatomy and physiology, chemistry, physics, microbiology, and mathematics. Technical courses deal with procedures, equipment, and clinical tests.

More than 40 States license respiratory care personnel. Aspiring respiratory care practitioners should check on licensure requirements with the board of respiratory care examiners for the State in which they plan to work.

The National Board for Respiratory Care (NBRC) offers voluntary certification and registration to graduates of CoARC-accredited programs. Two credentials are awarded to respiratory therapists who satisfy the requirements: Registered Respiratory Therapist (RRT) and Certified Respiratory Therapist (CRT). Graduates from 2- and 4-year programs in respiratory therapy may take the CRT examination. CRTs who meet education and experience requirements can take two separate examinations, leading to the award of the RRT. Either the CRT or RRT examination is the standard in the States requiring licensure.

Most employers require applicants for entry-level or generalist positions to hold the CRT or be eligible to take the certification examination. Supervisory positions and those in intensive care specialties usually require the RRT (or RRT eligibility). Therapists should be sensitive to patients' physical and psychological needs. Respiratory care practitioners must pay attention to detail, follow instructions, and work as part of a team. In addition, operating complicated equipment requires mechanical ability and manual dexterity.

High school students interested in a career in respiratory care should take courses in health, biology, mathematics, chemistry, and physics. Respiratory care involves basic mathematical problem solving and an understanding of chemical and physical principles. For example, respiratory care workers must be able to compute medication dosages and calculate gas concentrations.

Respiratory therapists advance in clinical practice by moving from care of general to critical patients who have significant problems in other organ systems, such as the heart or kidneys. Respiratory therapists, especially those with 4-year degrees, may also advance to supervisory or managerial positions in a respiratory therapy department. Respiratory therapists in home care and equipment rental firms may become branch managers. Some respiratory therapists advance by moving into teaching positions.

JOB OUTLOOK

Job opportunities are expected to remain good. Employment of respiratory therapists is expected to increase faster than the average for all occupations through the year 2010, because of substantial growth of the middle-aged and elderly population-a development that will heighten the incidence of cardiopulmonary disease.

Older Americans suffer most from respiratory ailments and cardiopulmonary diseases such as pneumonia, chronic bronchitis, emphysema, and heart disease. As their numbers increase, the need for respiratory therapists will increase, as well. In addition, advances in treating victims of heart attacks, accident victims, and premature infants (many of whom are dependent on a ventilator during part of their treatment) will increase the demand for the services of respiratory care practitioners. Opportunities are expected to be favorable for respiratory therapists with cardiopulmonary care skills and experience working with infants.

Although hospitals will continue to employ the vast majority of therapists, a growing number of therapists can expect to work outside of hospitals in respiratory therapy clinics, offices of physicians, nursing homes, or homecare.

EARNINGS

Median annual earnings of respiratory therapists were $37,680 in 2000. The middle 50 percent earned between $32,140 and $43,430. The lowest 10 percent earned less than $28,620, and the highest 10 percent earned more than $50,660. In hospitals, median annual earnings of respiratory therapists were $38,040 in 2000. Median annual earnings of respiratory therapy technicians were $32,860 in 2000. The middle 50 percent earned between $27,280 and $39,740. The lowest 10 percent earned less than $22,830, and the highest 10 percent earned more than $46,800. Median annual earnings of respiratory therapy technicians employed in hospitals were $32,830 in 2000.

RELATED OCCUPATIONS

Respiratory therapists, under the supervision of a physician, administer respiratory care and life support to patients with heart and lung difficulties. Other workers who care for, treat, or train people to improve their physical condition include registered nurses, occupational therapists, physical therapists, and radiation therapists.

SOURCES OF ADDITIONAL INFORMATION

Information concerning a career in respiratory care is available from: American Association for Respiratory Care, 11030 Ables Lane, Dallas, TX 75229-4593. Internet: http://www.aarc.org

For the current list of CoARC-accredited educational programs for respiratory care practitioners, write to: Committee on Accreditation for Respiratory Care, 1248 Harwood Rd., Bedford, TX 76021-4244. Internet: http://www.coarc.com

Information on gaining credentials in respiratory care and a list of State licensing agencies can be obtained from: The National Board for Respiratory Care, Inc., 8310 Nieman Rd., Lenexa, KS 66214-1579.

Chapter 14

SPEECH-LANGUAGE PATHOLOGISTS AND AUDIOLOGISTS

SIGNIFICANT POINTS

- Employment of speech-language pathologists and audiologists is expected to grow rapidly because the growing population in older age groups is prone to medical conditions that result in hearing and speech problems.
- About half work in schools, and most others are employed by healthcare facilities.
- A master's degree in speech-language pathology or audiology is the standard credential.

NATURE OF THE WORK

Speech-language pathologists assess, diagnose, treat, and help to prevent speech, language, cognitive, communication, voice, swallowing, fluency, and other related disorders; audiologists identify, assess, and manage auditory, balance, and other neural systems. Speech-language pathologists work with people who cannot make speech sounds, or cannot make them clearly; those with speech rhythm and fluency problems, such as stuttering; people with voice quality problems, such as inappropriate pitch or harsh voice; those with problems understanding and producing language; those who wish to improve their communication skills by modifying an accent; and those with cognitive communication impairments, such as attention, memory, and problem solving disorders. They also work with people who have oral motor problems causing eating and swallowing difficulties.

Speech and language problems can result from a variety of problems including hearing loss, brain injury or deterioration, cerebral palsy, stroke, cleft palate, voice pathology, mental retardation, or emotional problems. Problems can be congenital, developmental, or acquired.

Speech-language pathologists use written and oral tests, as well as special instruments, to diagnose the nature and extent of impairment and to record and analyze speech, language, and swallowing irregularities. Speech-language pathologists develop an individualized plan of care, tailored to each patient's needs. For individuals with little or no speech capability, speech-language pathologists may select augmentative or alternative communication methods, including automated devices and sign language, and teach their use. They teach these individuals how to make sounds, improve their voices, or increase their language skills to communicate more effectively. Speech-language pathologists help patients develop, or recover, reliable communication skills so patients can fulfill their educational, vocational, and social roles. Most speech-language pathologists provide direct clinical services to individuals with communication or swallowing disorders.

In speech and language clinics, they may independently develop and carry out treatment programs. In medical facilities, they may work with physicians, social workers, psychologists, and other therapists. Speech-language pathologists in schools develop individual or group programs, counsel parents, and may assist teachers with classroom activities. Speech-language pathologists keep records on the initial evaluation, progress, and discharge of clients. This helps pinpoint problems, tracks client progress, and justifies the cost of treatment when applying for reimbursement. They counsel individuals and their families concerning communication disorders and how to cope with the stress and misunderstanding that often accompany them. They also work with family members to recognize and change behavior patterns that impede communication and treatment and show them communication-enhancing techniques to use at home. Some speech-language pathologists conduct research on how people communicate. Others design and develop equipment or techniques for diagnosing and treating speech problems.

Audiologists work with people who have hearing, balance, and related problems. They use audiometers, computers, and other testing devices to measure the loudness at which a person begins to hear sounds, the ability to distinguish between sounds, and the nature and extent of hearing loss. Audiologists interpret these results and may coordinate them with medical, educational, and psychological information to make a diagnosis and determine a course of treatment.

Hearing disorders can result from a variety of causes including trauma at birth, viral infections, genetic disorders, exposure to loud noise, or aging. Treatment may include examining and cleaning the ear canal, fitting and dispensing hearing aids or other assistive devices, and audiologic rehabilitation (including auditory training or instruction in speech or lip reading). Audiologists may recommend, fit, and dispense personal or large area amplification systems, such as hearing aids and alerting devices. Audiologists provide fitting and tuning of cochlear implants and provide the necessary rehabilitation for adjustment to listening with implant amplification systems. They also measure noise levels in workplaces and conduct hearing protection programs in industry, as well as in schools and communities. Audiologists provide direct clinical services to individuals with hearing or balance disorders. In audiology (hearing) clinics, they may independently develop and carry out treatment programs.

Audiologists, in a variety of settings, work as members of interdisciplinary professional teams in planning and implementing service delivery for children and adults, from birth to old age. Similar to speech-language pathologists, audiologists keep records on the initial evaluation, progress, and discharge of clients. These records help pinpoint problems, track client progress, and justify the cost of treatment, when applying for reimbursement. Audiologists may conduct research on types of, and treatment for, hearing, balance, and related disorders. Others design and develop equipment or techniques for diagnosing and treating these disorders.

WORKING CONDITIONS

Speech-language pathologists and audiologists usually work at a desk or table in clean comfortable surroundings. The job is not physically demanding but does require attention to detail and intense concentration. The emotional needs of clients and their families may be demanding. Most full-time speech-language pathologists and audiologists work about 40 hours per week; some work part time. Those who work on a contract basis may spend a substantial amount of time traveling between facilities.

EMPLOYMENT

Speech-language pathologists and audiologists held about 101,000 jobs in 2000. Speech-language pathologists held about 88,000 jobs; and audiologists held about 13,000. About one-half of jobs for speech-language pathologists and audiologists were in preschools, elementary and secondary schools, or colleges and universities. Others were in offices of speech-language pathologists and audiologists; hospitals; offices of physicians; speech, language, and hearing centers; home health agencies; or other facilities.

Audiologists are more likely to be employed in independent healthcare offices, while speech-language pathologists are more likely to work in school settings. A small number of speech-language pathologists and audiologists are self-employed in private practice. They contract to provide services in schools, physician's offices, hospitals, or nursing homes, or work as consultants to industry.

TRAINING, OTHER QUALIFICATIONS AND ADVANCEMENT

Of the States that regulate licensing (45 for speech-language pathologists and 47 for audiologists), almost all require a master's degree or equivalent. Other requirements are 300 to 375 hours of supervised clinical experience, a passing score on a national examination, and 9 months of postgraduate professional clinical experience. Forty-one States have continuing education requirements for licensure renewal. Medicaid, medicare, and private health insurers generally require a practitioner to be licensed to qualify for reimbursement.

About 242 colleges and universities offer graduate programs in speech-language pathology. Courses cover anatomy and physiology of the areas of the body involved in speech, language, and hearing; the development of normal speech, language, and hearing; the nature of disorders; acoustics; and psychological aspects of communication. Graduate students also learn to evaluate and treat speech, language, and hearing disorders and receive supervised clinical training in communication disorders.

About 112 colleges and universities offer graduate programs in audiology in the United States. Course work includes anatomy; physiology; basic science; math; physics; genetics; normal and abnormal communication development; auditory, balance and neural systems assessment and treatment; audiologic rehabilitation; and ethics.

Speech-language pathologists can acquire the Certificate of Clinical Competence in Speech-Language Pathology (CCC-SLP) offered by the American Speech-Language-Hearing Association, and audiologists can earn the Certificate of Clinical Competence in Audiology (CCC-A). To earn a CCC, a person must have a graduate degree and 375 hours of supervised clinical experience, complete a 36-week postgraduate clinical fellowship, and pass a written examination.

According to the American Speech-Language-Hearing Association, as of 2007, audiologists will need to have a bachelor's degree and complete 75 hours of credit toward a doctoral degree in order to seek certification. As of 2012, audiologists will have to earn a doctoral degree in order to be certified.

Speech-language pathologists and audiologists should be able to effectively communicate diagnostic test results, diagnoses, and proposed treatment in a manner easily understood by their clients. They must be able to approach problems objectively and provide support to clients and their families. Because a client's progress may be slow, patience, compassion, and good listening skills are necessary.

JOB OUTLOOK

Employment of speech-language pathologists and audiologists is expected to grow much faster than the average for all occupations through the year 2010. Because hearing loss is strongly associated with aging, rapid growth in the population age 55 and over will cause the number of persons with hearing impairment to increase markedly. In addition, baby boomers are now entering middle age, when the possibility of neurological disorders and associated speech, language, and hearing impairments increases. Medical advances are also improving the survival rate of premature infants and trauma and stroke victims, who then need assessment and possible treatment.

In health services facilities, Federal legislation imposing limits on reimbursement for therapy services may adversely affect the job market for therapy providers over the near term. Employment in schools will increase along with growth in elementary and secondary school enrollments, including enrollment of special education students. Federal law guarantees special education and related services to all eligible children with disabilities. Greater awareness of the importance of early identification and diagnosis of speech, language, and hearing disorders will also increase employment.

The number of speech-language pathologists and audiologists in private practice will rise due to the increasing use of contract services by hospitals, schools, and nursing homes. In addition to job openings stemming from employment growth, some openings for speech-language pathologists and audiologists will arise from the need to replace those who leave the occupation.

EARNINGS

Median annual earnings of speech-language pathologists were $46,640 in 2000. The middle 50 percent earned between $37,670 and $56,980. The lowest 10 percent earned less than $30,720, and the highest 10 percent earned more than $69,980. Median annual earnings in the industries employing the largest numbers of speech-language pathologists in 2000 were as follows:

- Hospitals $49,960
- Offices of other health practitioners $47,170
- Elementary and secondary schools $43,710

Median annual earnings of audiologists were $44,830 in 2000. The middle 50 percent earned between $37,000 and $55,290. The lowest 10 percent earned less than $30,850, and the highest 10 percent earned more than $68,570. According to a 2000 survey by the American Speech-Language-Hearing Association, the median annual salary for full-time certified speech-language pathologists who worked 11 or 12 months annually was $44,000; for audiologists, $48,000. For those who worked 9 or 10 months annually, the median annual salary for speech-language pathologists was $41,000; for audiologists, $45,000. Speech-language pathologists with doctorate degrees who worked 11 or 12 months annually earned $62,500; and audiologists, $70,000.

RELATED OCCUPATIONS

Speech-language pathologists and audiologists specialize in the prevention, diagnosis, and treatment of speech and language and hearing problems. Workers in related occupations include occupational therapists, optometrists, physical therapists, psychologists, recreational therapists, and rehabilitation counselors.

SOURCES OF ADDITIONAL INFORMATION

State licensing boards can provide information on licensure requirements. State departments of education can supply information on certification requirements for those who wish to work in public schools.

General information on careers in speech-language pathology and audiology is available from: American Speech-Language-Hearing Association, 10801 Rockville Pike, Rockville, MD 20852. Internet: http://professional.asha.org

Information on a career in audiology is also available from: American Academy of Audiology, 8201 Greensboro Dr., Suite 300, McLean, VA 22102.

Chapter 15

VETERINARIANS

SIGNIFICANT POINTS

- Graduation from an accredited college of veterinary medicine and a license to practice are required.
- Competition for admission to veterinary school is keen.

NATURE OF THE WORK

Veterinarians play a major role in the healthcare of pets, livestock, and zoo, sporting, and laboratory animals. Some veterinarians use their skills to protect humans against diseases carried by animals and conduct clinical research on human and animal health problems. Others work in basic research, broadening the scope of fundamental theoretical knowledge, and in applied research, developing new ways to use knowledge. Most veterinarians perform clinical work in private practices.

More than one-half of these veterinarians predominately, or exclusively, treat small animals. Small animal practitioners usually care for companion animals, such as dogs and cats, but also treat birds, reptiles, rabbits, and other animals that can be kept as pets. Some veterinarians work in mixed animal practices where they see pigs, goats, sheep, and some nondomestic animals, in addition to companion animals.

Veterinarians in clinical practice diagnose animal health problems; vaccinate against diseases, such as distemper and rabies; medicate animals suffering from infections or illnesses; treat and dress wounds; set fractures;

perform surgery; and advise owners about animal feeding, behavior, and breeding.

A small number of private practice veterinarians work exclusively with large animals, focusing mostly on horses or cows but may also care for various kinds of food animals. These veterinarians usually drive to farms or ranches to provide veterinary services for herds or individual animals. Much of this work involves preventive care to maintain the health of the food animals. These veterinarians test for and vaccinate against diseases and consult with farm or ranch owners and managers on animal production, feeding, and housing issues. They also treat and dress wounds, set fractures, and perform surgery-including cesarean sections on birthing animals.

Veterinarians also euthanize animals when necessary. Other veterinarians care for zoo, aquarium, or laboratory animals. Veterinarians who treat animals use medical equipment, such as stethoscopes; surgical instruments; and diagnostic equipment, such as radiographic and ultra-sound equipment. Veterinarians working in research use a full range of sophisticated laboratory equipment. Veterinarians can contribute to human as well as animal health. A number of veterinarians work with physicians and scientists as they research ways to prevent and treat human health problems, such as cancer, AIDS, and alcohol or drug abuse. Some determine the effects of drug therapies, antibiotics, or new surgical techniques by testing them on animals. Some veterinarians are involved in food safety at various levels.

Veterinarians who are livestock inspectors check animals for transmissible diseases, advise owners on treatment, and may quarantine animals. Veterinarians who are meat, poultry, or egg product inspectors examine slaughtering and processing plants, check live animals and carcasses for disease, and enforce government regulations regarding food purity and sanitation.

WORKING CONDITIONS

Veterinarians often work long hours, with well over one-third of full-time workers spending 50 or more hours on the job. Those in group practices may take turns being on call for evening, night, or weekend work; and solo practitioners can work extended and weekend hours, responding to emergencies or squeezing in unexpected appointments. Veterinarians in large animal practice also spend time driving between their office and farms or ranches. They work outdoors in all kinds of weather, and have to treat animals or perform surgery under less-than-sanitary conditions. When working with animals that are frightened or in pain, veterinarians risk being bitten, kicked, or scratched.

Veterinarians working in non-clinical areas, such as public health and research, have working conditions similar to those of other professionals in those lines of work. In these cases, veterinarians enjoy clean, well lit offices or laboratories and spend much of their time dealing with people rather than animals.

EMPLOYMENT

Veterinarians held about 59,000 jobs in 2000. About 28 percent were self-employed in solo or group practices. Most others were employees of another veterinary practice. The Federal Government employed about 800 civilian veterinarians, chiefly in the U.S. Departments of Agriculture and Health and Human Services. Other employers of veterinarians are State and local governments, colleges of veterinary medicine, medical schools, research laboratories, animal food companies, and pharmaceutical companies. A few veterinarians work for zoos; but most veterinarians caring for zoo animals are private practitioners who contract with zoos to provide services, usually on a part-time basis.

TRAINING, OTHER QUALIFICATIONS AND ADVANCEMENT

Prospective veterinarians must graduate from a 4-year program at an accredited college of veterinary medicine with a Doctor of Veterinary Medicine (D.V.M. or V.M.D.) degree and obtain a license to practice. There are 27 colleges in 26 States that meet accreditation standards set by the Council on Education of the American Veterinary Medical Association. The prerequisites for admission vary by veterinary medical college. Many of these colleges do not require a bachelor's degree for entrance; but all require a significant number of credit hours-ranging from 45 to 90 semester hours-at the undergraduate level. However, most of the students admitted have completed an undergraduate program.

Preveterinary courses emphasize the sciences; and veterinary medical colleges typically require classes in organic and inorganic chemistry, physics, biochemistry, general biology, animal biology, animal nutrition, genetics, vertebrate embryology, cellular biology, microbiology, zoology, and systemic physiology. Some programs require calculus; some require only statistics, college algebra and trigonometry, or precalculus; and others require no math at all. Most veterinary medical colleges also require core courses, including some in English or literature, the social sciences, and the humanities. Most veterinary medical colleges will only consider applicants who have a minimum grade point average (GPA). The required GPA varies by school, from a low of 2.5 to a high of 3.2, based on a maximum GPA of 4.0. However, the average GPA of candidates at most schools is higher than these minimums. Those who receive offers of admission usually have a GPA of 3.0 or better. In addition to satisfying preveterinary course requirements, applicants must also submit test scores from the Graduate Record Examination (GRE), the Veterinary College Admission Test (VCAT), or the Medical College Admission Test (MCAT), depending on the preference of each college.

Additionally, in the admissions process, veterinary medical colleges weigh heavily a candidate's veterinary and animal experience. Formal experience, such as work with veterinarians or scientists in clinics, agribusiness, research, or in some area of health science, is particularly advantageous. Less formal experience, such as working with animals on a farm or ranch or at a stable or animal shelter, is also helpful. Students must demonstrate ambition and an eagerness to work with animals. Competition for admission to veterinary school is keen. The number of accredited veterinary colleges has remained at 27 since 1983, whereas the number of applicants has risen. About 1 in 3 applicants was accepted in 1998. Most veterinary medical colleges are public, State-supported institutions and reserve the majority of their openings for in-state residents.

Twenty-one States that do not have a veterinary medical college agree to pay a fee or subsidy to help cover the cost of veterinary education for a limited number of their residents at one or more out-of-state colleges. Nonresident students who are admitted under such a contract may have to pay out-of-state tuition, or they may have to repay their State of residency all, or part, of the subsidy provided to the contracting college. Residents of the remaining 3 States (Connecticut, Maine, and Vermont) and the District of Columbia may apply to any of the 27 veterinary medical colleges as an at-large applicant. The number of positions available to at-large applicants is very limited at most schools, making admission difficult.

While in veterinary medical college, students receive additional academic instruction in the basic sciences for the first 2 years. Later in the program, students are exposed to clinical procedures, such as diagnosing and treating animal diseases and performing surgery. They also do laboratory work in anatomy, biochemistry, medicine, and other scientific subjects. At most veterinary medical colleges, students who plan a career in research can earn both a D.V.M degree and a Doctor of Philosophy (Ph.D.) degree at the same time. Veterinary graduates who plan to work with specific types of animals or specialize in a clinical area, such as pathology, surgery, radiology, or laboratory animal medicine, usually complete a 1-year internship. Interns receive a small salary but usually find that their internship experience leads to a higher beginning salary, relative to other starting veterinarians.

Veterinarians who seek board certification in a specialty must also complete a 2- to 3-year residency program that provides intensive training in specialties, such as internal medicine, oncology, radiology, surgery, dermatology, anesthesiology, neurology, cardiology, ophthalmology, and exotic small animal medicine. All States and the District of Columbia require that veterinarians be licensed before they can practice. The only exemptions are for veterinarians working for some Federal agencies and some State governments. Licensing is controlled by the States and is not strictly uniform, although all States require successful completion of the D.V.M. degree-or equivalent education-and passage of a national board examination.

The Educational Commission for Foreign Veterinary Graduates (ECFVG) grants certification to individuals trained outside the U.S. who demonstrate that they meet specified requirements for the English language and clinical proficiency. ECFVG certification fulfills the educational requirement for licensure in all States except Nebraska. Applicants for licensure satisfy the examination requirement by passing the North American Veterinary Licensing Exam (NAVLE), which recently replaced the National Board Examination (NBE) and the Clinical Competency Test (CCT). The new NAVLE, administered on computer, takes one day to complete and consists of 360 multiple- choice questions, covering all aspects of veterinary medicine. The NAVLE also includes visual materials designed to test diagnostic skills.

The majority of States also require candidates to pass a State jurisprudence examination covering State laws and regulations. Some States also do additional testing on clinical competency. There are few reciprocal agreements between States, making it difficult for a veterinarian to practice in a different State without first taking another State examination. Forty-one States have continuing education requirements for licensed veterinarians. Requirements differ by State and may involve attending a class or otherwise demonstrating knowledge of recent medical and veterinary advances. Most veterinarians begin as employees or partners in established practices. Despite the substantial financial investment in equipment, office space, and staff, many veterinarians with experience set up their own practice or purchase an established one. Newly trained veterinarians can become U.S. Government meat and poultry inspectors, disease-control workers, epidemiologists, research assistants, or commissioned officers in the U.S. Public Health Service, U.S. Army, or U.S. Air Force. A State license may be required. Prospective veterinarians must have good manual dexterity. They should have an affinity for animals and the ability to get along with animal owners. Additionally, they should be able to quickly make decisions in emergencies.

JOB OUTLOOK

Employment of veterinarians is expected to grow faster than the average for all occupations through the year 2010. Job openings stemming from the need to replace veterinarians who retire or otherwise leave the labor force will be almost as numerous as new jobs resulting from employment growth over the 2000-10 period. Most veterinarians practice in animal hospitals or clinics and care primarily for companion animals. The number of dogs as pets is expected to increase more slowly during the projection period than in the previous decade. However, faster growth of the cat population is expected to increase the demand for feline medicine and veterinary services, offsetting any reduced demand for veterinary care for dogs. Also, as non-necessity income generally increases with age, those who own pets may be more inclined to seek veterinary services. Small increases in the total number of household pets, coupled with the movement of baby boomers into the 34 to 59 year age group, means that the willingness by pet owners to pay for veterinary services should continue. In addition, pet owners are becoming more aware of the availability of advanced care and may increasingly take advantage of nontraditional veterinary services, such as preventive dental care, and may more willingly pay for - intensive care than in the past. Finally, new technologies and medical advancements should permit veterinarians to offer better care to animals. New graduates continue to be attracted to small animal medicine because they prefer to deal with pets and to live and work near highly populated areas. This situation will not necessarily limit the ability of veterinarians to find employment or to set up and maintain a practice in a particular area. Rather, beginning veterinarians may take positions requiring evening or weekend work to accommodate the extended hours of operation that many practices are offering. Some veterinarians take salaried positions in retail stores offering veterinary services. Self-employed veterinarians usually have to work hard and long to build a sufficient client base. The number of jobs for large animal veterinarians is expected to grow slowly, because productivity gains in the agricultural production industry mean demand for fewer veterinarians than before to treat food animals. Nevertheless, job prospects may be better for veterinarians who specialize in farm animals than for small animal practitioners, because most veterinary medical college graduates do not have the desire to work in rural or isolated areas. Continued support for public health and food safety, international and national disease control programs, and biomedical research on human health problems will contribute to the demand for veterinarians, although such positions are few in number. However, anticipated budget tightening in the Federal Government may lead to low funding levels for some programs, limiting job growth. Veterinarians with training in public health and epidemiology should have the best opportunities for a career in the Federal Government.

EARNINGS

Median annual earnings of veterinarians were $60,910 in 2000. The middle 50 percent earned between $47,020 and $84,220. The lowest 10 percent earned less than $36,670, and the highest 10 percent earned more than $128,720. According to a survey by the American Veterinary Medical Association, average starting salaries of 2000 veterinary medical college graduates varied by type of practice as follows:

- Small animal, predominant $42,918
- Small animal, exclusive $42,640
- Large animal, exclusive $41,629
- Large animal, predominant $41,439
- Mixed animal $40,358
- Equine $28,526

New veterinary medical college graduates who enter the Federal Government usually start at $35,808. Beginning salaries were slightly higher in selected areas where the prevailing local pay level was higher. The average annual salary for veterinarians in the Federal Government in nonsupervisory, supervisory, and managerial positions was $ 67,482 in 2001.

RELATED OCCUPATIONS

Veterinarians prevent, diagnose, and treat diseases, disorders, and injuries in animals. Those who do similar work for humans include chiropractors, dentists, optometrists, physicians and surgeons, and podiatrists. Veterinarians have extensive training in physical and life sciences, and some do scientific and medical research, closely paralleling occupation biological and medical scientists. Animal care and service workers and veterinary technologists, technicians and assistants work extensively with animals. Like veterinarians, they must have patience and feel comfortable with animals. However, the level of training required for these occupations is substantially less than that needed by veterinarians.

SOURCES OF ADDITIONAL INFORMATION

For additional information on careers in veterinary medicine and a list of U.S. schools and colleges of veterinary medicine and accreditation policies, send a letter-size, self- addressed, stamped envelope to: American Veterinary Medical Association, 1931 N. Meacham Rd., Suite 100, Schaumburg, IL 60173-4360. Internet: http://www.avma.org

For information on veterinary education, write to: Association of American Veterinary Medical Colleges, 1101 Vermont Ave. NW., Suite 710, Washington, DC 20005. Internet: http://www.aavmc.org

For information on scholarships, grants, and loans, contact the financial aid officer at the veterinary schools to which you wish to apply.

Chapter 16

CARDIOVASCULAR TECHNOLOGISTS AND TECHNICIANS

SIGNIFICANT POINTS

- Employment will grow faster than the average, but the number of job openings created will be low, because the occupation is small.
- Job prospects will be good due to an aging population and increased need for vascular technology and sonography as an alternative for more costly and invasive heart surgery.
- About 7 out of 10 jobs are in hospitals, in both inpatient and outpatient settings.

NATURE OF THE WORK

Cardiovascular technologists and technicians assist physicians in diagnosing and treating cardiac (heart) and peripheral vascular (blood vessel) ailments. Cardiovascular technologists may specialize in three areas of practice: Invasive cardiology, echocardiography, and vascular technology. Cardiovascular technicians who specialize in electrocardiograms (EKGs), stress testing, and Holter monitors are known as cardiographic or EKG technicians. Cardiovascular technologists specializing in invasive procedures are called cardiology technologists. They assist physicians with cardiac catheterization procedures in which a small tube, or catheter, is wound through a patient's blood vessel from a spot on the patient's leg into the heart.

The procedure can determine if a blockage exists in the blood vessels that supply the heart muscle and help diagnose other problems. Part of the procedure may involve balloon angioplasty, which can be used to treat blockages of blood vessels or heart valves, without the need for heart surgery. Cardiology technologists assist physicians as they insert a catheter with a balloon on the end to the point of the obstruction. Technologists prepare patients for cardiac catheterization and balloon angioplasty by first positioning them on an examining table and then shaving, cleaning, and administering anesthesia to the top of the patient's leg near the groin. During the procedures, they monitor patients' blood pressure and heart rate using EKG equipment and notify the physician if something appears wrong. Technologists also may prepare and monitor patients during open-heart surgery and the implantation of pacemakers. Cardiovascular technologists who specialize in echocardiography or vascular technology often run noninvasive tests using ultra- sound instrumentation, such as doppler ultrasound. Tests are called "noninvasive" if they do not require the insertion of probes or other instruments into the patient's body. The ultrasound instrumentation transmits high frequency sound waves into areas of the patient's body and then processes reflected echoes of the sound waves to form an image. Technologists view the ultrasound image on a screen that may be recorded on videotape or photographed for interpretation and diagnosis by a physician. While performing the scan, technologists check the image on the screen for subtle differences between healthy and diseased areas, decide which images to include, and judge if the images are satisfactory for diagnostic purposes. They also explain the procedure to patients, record additional medical history, select appropriate equipment settings, and change the patient's position as necessary. Those who assist physicians in the diagnosis of disorders affecting circulation are known as vascular technologists or vascular sonographers. They perform a medical history and evaluate pulses by listening to the sounds of the arteries for abnormalities. Then they perform a noninvasive procedure using ultrasound instrumentation to record vascular information, such as vascular blood flow, blood pressure, limb volume changes, oxygen saturation, cerebral circulation, peripheral circulation, and abdominal circulation. Many of these tests are performed during or immediately after surgery. Technologists who use ultrasound to examine the heart chambers, valves, and vessels are referred to as cardiac sonographers, or echocardiographers. They use ultrasound instrumentation to create images called echocardiograms. This may be done while the patient is either resting or physically active. Technologists may administer medication to a physically active patient to assess their heart function. Cardiac sonographers may also assist physicians who perform transesophageal echocardiography, which involves placing a tube in the patient's esophagus to obtain ultrasound images. Cardiovascular technicians who obtain EKGs are known as electrocardiograph (or EKG) technicians. To take a basic EKG, which traces electrical impulses transmitted by the heart, technicians attach electrodes to the patient's chest, arms, and legs, and then manipulate switches on an EKG machine to obtain a reading. A printout is made for interpretation by the physician. This test is done before most kinds of surgery and as part of a routine physical examination, especially for persons who have reached middle age or have a history of cardiovascular problems. EKG technicians with advanced training perform Holter monitor and stress testing. For Holter monitoring, technicians place electrodes on the patient's chest and attach a portable EKG monitor to the patient's belt. Following 24 or more hours of normal activity for the patient, the technician removes a tape from the monitor and places it in a scanner. After checking the quality of the recorded impulses on an electronic screen, the technician usually prints the information from the tape so that a physician can interpret it later. Physicians use the output from the scanner to diagnose heart ailments, such as heart rhythm abnormalities or problems with pacemakers. For a treadmill stress test, EKG technicians document the patient's medical history, explain the procedure, connect the patient to an EKG monitor, and obtain a baseline reading and resting blood pressure. Next, they monitor the heart's performance while the patient is walking on a treadmill, gradually increasing the treadmill's speed to observe the effect of increased exertion. Like vascular technologists and cardiac sonographers, cardiographic technicians who perform EKG, Holter monitor, and stress tests are known as "noninvasive" technicians. Some cardiovascular technologists and technicians schedule appointments, type doctor interpretations, maintain patient files, and care for equipment.

WORKING CONDITIONS

Technologists and technicians generally work a 5-day, 40-hour week that may include weekends. Those in catheterization labs tend to work longer hours and may work evenings. They also may be on call during the night and on weekends. Cardiovascular technologists and technicians spend a lot of time walking and standing. Those who work in catheterization labs may face stressful working conditions, because they are in close contact with patients with serious heart ailments. Some patients, for example, may encounter complications from time to time that have life or death implications.

EMPLOYMENT

Cardiovascular technologists and technicians held about 39,000 jobs in 2000. Most worked in hospital cardiology departments, whereas some worked in offices of cardiologists or other physicians, cardiac rehabilitation centers, or ambulatory surgery centers.

TRAINING, OTHER QUALIFICATIONS AND ADVANCEMENT

Although a few cardiovascular technologists, vascular technologists, and cardiac sonographers are currently trained on the job, most receive training in 2- to 4-year programs. Cardiovascular technologists, vascular technologists, and cardiac sonographers normally complete a 2-year junior or community college program. One year is dedicated to core courses followed by a year of specialized instruction in either invasive, noninvasive cardiovascular, or noninvasive vascular technology. Those who are qualified in a related allied health profession only need to complete the year of specialized instruction. Graduates from the 23 programs accredited by the Joint Review Committee on Education in Cardiovascular Technology are eligible to obtain professional certification through Cardiovascular Credentialing International in cardiac catheterization, echocardiography, vascular ultrasound, and cardiographic techniques. Cardiac sonographers and vascular technologists may also obtain certification with the American Registry of Diagnostic Medical Sonographers. For basic EKGs, Holter monitoring, and stress testing, 1-year certificate programs exist; but most EKG technicians are still trained on the job by an EKG supervisor or a cardiologist. On-the-job training usually lasts about 8 to 16 weeks. Most employers prefer to train people already in the health care field-nursing aides, for example. Some EKG technicians are students enrolled in 2-year programs to become technologists, working part-time to gain experience and make contact with employers. Cardiovascular technologists and technicians must be reliable, have mechanical aptitude, and be able to follow detailed instructions. A pleasant, relaxed manner for putting patients at ease is an asset.

JOB OUTLOOK

Employment of cardiovascular technologists and technicians is expected to grow faster than the average for all occupations through the year 2010. Growth will occur as the population ages, because older people have a higher incidence of heart problems. Employment of vascular technologists and echocardiographers will grow as advances in vascular technology and sonography reduce the need for more costly and invasive procedures. Employment of EKG technicians is expected to decline, as hospitals train nursing aides and others to perform basic EKG procedures. Individuals trained in Holter monitoring and stress testing are expected to have more favorable job prospects than those who can only perform a basic EKG. Some job openings for cardiovascular technologists and technicians will arise from replacement needs, as individuals transfer to other jobs or leave the labor force. Relatively few job openings, due to both growth and replacement needs are expected, however, because the occupation is small.

EARNINGS

Median annual earnings of cardiovascular technologists and technicians were $33,350 in 2000. The middle 50 percent earned between $24,590 and $43,450. The lowest 10 percent earned less than $19,540, and the highest 10 percent earned more than $52,930. Median annual earnings of cardiovascular technologists and technicians in 2000 were $33,100 in offices and clinics of medical doctors and $32,860 in hospitals.

RELATED OCCUPATIONS

Cardiovascular technologists and technicians operate sophisticated equipment that helps physicians and other health practitioners diagnose and treat patients. So do diagnostic medical sonographers, nuclear medicine technologists, radiation therapists, radiologic technologists and technicians, and respiratory therapists.

SOURCES OF ADDITIONAL INFORMATION

For general information about a career in cardiovascular technology, contact: Alliance of Cardiovascular Professionals, 4456 Corporation Ln., Suite 165, Virginia Beach, VA 23462. Internet: http://www.acp-online.org/index.html

For a list of accredited programs in cardiovascular technology, contact: Joint Review Committee on Education in Cardiovascular Technology, 3525 Ellicott Mills Dr., Suite N, Ellicott City, MD 21043-4547. Internet: http://www.sicp.com/jrc-cvt

For information on vascular technology, contact: The Society of Vascular Technology, 4601 Presidents Dr., Suite 260, Lanham, MD 20706-4365. Internet: http://www.svtnet.org

For information on echocardiography, contact: American Society of Echocardiography, 4101 Lake Boone Trail, Suite 201, Raleigh, NC 27607. Internet: http://www.asecho.org

For information regarding registration and certification, contact:

- Cardiovascular Credentialing International, 4456 Corporation Lane, Suite 110, Virginia Beach, VA 23462. Internet: http://www.cci-online.org
- American Registry of Diagnostic Medical Sonographers, 600 Jefferson Plaza, Suite 360, Rockville, MD 20852-1150. Internet: http://www.ardms.org

Chapter 17

CLINICAL LABORATORY TECHNOLOGISTS AND TECHNICIANS

SIGNIFICANT POINTS

- Clinical laboratory technologists usually have a bachelor's degree with a major in medical technology or in one of the life sciences; clinical laboratory technicians need either an associate's degree or a certificate.
- Employment is expected to grow as fast as average as the volume of laboratory tests increases with population growth and the development of new types of tests.

NATURE OF THE WORK

Clinical laboratory testing plays a crucial role in the detection, diagnosis, and treatment of disease. Clinical laboratory technologists, also referred to as clinical laboratory scientists or medical technologists, and clinical laboratory technicians, also known as medical technicians or medical laboratory technicians, perform most of these tests. Clinical laboratory personnel examine and analyze body fluids, tissues, and cells. They look for bacteria, parasites, and other microorganisms; analyze the chemical content of fluids; match blood for transfusions; and test for drug levels in the blood to show how a patient is responding to treatment. These technologists also prepare specimens for examination, count cells, and look for abnormal cells.

They use automated equipment and instruments capable of performing a number of tests simultaneously, as well as microscopes, cell counters, and other sophisticated laboratory equipment. Then, they analyze the results and relay them to physicians. With - increasing automation and the use of computer technology, the work of technologists and technicians has become less hands-on and more analytical. The complexity of tests performed, the level of judgment needed, and the amount of responsibility workers assume depend largely on the amount of education and experience they have. Medical and clinical laboratory technologists generally have a bachelor's degree in medical technology or in one of the life sciences, or they have a combination of formal training and work experience. They perform complex chemical, biological, hematological, immunologic, microscopic, and bacteriological tests. Technologists microscopically examine blood, tissue, and other body substances. They make cultures of body fluid and tissue samples, to determine the presence of bacteria, fungi, parasites, or other microorganisms. They analyze samples for chemical content or reaction and determine blood glucose and cholesterol levels. They also type and cross match blood samples for transfusions. Medical and clinical laboratory technologists evaluate test results, develop and modify procedures, and establish and monitor programs, to ensure the accuracy of tests. Some medical and clinical laboratory technologists supervise medical and clinical laboratory technicians. Technologists in small laboratories perform many types of tests, whereas those in large laboratories generally specialize. Technologists who prepare specimens and analyze the chemical and hormonal contents of body fluids are clinical chemistry technologists. Those who examine and identify bacteria and other microorganisms are microbiology technologists. Blood bank technologists, or immunohematology technologists, collect, type, and prepare blood and its components for transfusions. Immunology technologists examine elements and responses of the human immune system to foreign bodies. Cytotechnologists prepare slides of body cells and microscopically examine these cells for abnormalities that may signal the beginning of a cancerous growth. Molecular biology technologists perform complex genetic testing on cell samples. Medical and clinical laboratory technicians perform less complex tests and laboratory procedures than technologists. Technicians may prepare specimens and operate automated analyzers, for example, or they may perform manual tests following detailed instructions. Like technologists, they may work in several areas of the clinical laboratory or specialize in just one. Histology technicians cut and stain tissue specimens for microscopic examination by pathologists, and phlebotomists collect blood samples. They usually work under the supervision of medical and clinical laboratory technologists or laboratory managers.

WORKING CONDITIONS

Hours and other working conditions of clinical laboratory technologists and technicians vary, according to the size and type of employment setting. In large hospitals or in independent laboratories that operate continuously, personnel usually work the day, evening, or night shift and may work weekends and holidays. Laboratory personnel in small facilities may work on rotating shifts, rather than on a regular shift. In some facilities, laboratory personnel are on call several nights a week or on weekends, in case of an emergency. Clinical laboratory personnel are trained to work with infectious specimens. When proper methods of infection control and sterilization are followed, few hazards exist. Protective masks, gloves, and goggles are often necessary to ensure the safety of laboratory personnel. Laboratories usually are well-lighted and clean; however, specimens, solutions, and reagents used in the laboratory sometimes produce fumes. Laboratory workers may spend a great deal of time on their feet.

EMPLOYMENT

Clinical laboratory technologists and technicians held about 295,000 jobs in 2000. About half worked in hospitals. Most of the remaining jobs were found in medical laboratories or offices and clinics of physicians. A small number were in blood banks, research and testing laboratories, and in the Federal Government-at U.S. Department of Veterans Affairs hospitals and U.S. Public Health Service facilities.

TRAINING, OTHER QUALIFICATIONS AND ADVANCEMENT

The usual requirement for an entry-level position as a medical or clinical laboratory technologist is a bachelor's degree with a major in medical technology or in one of the life sciences. Universities and hospitals offer medical technology programs. It also is possible to qualify through a combination of education, on-the-job, and specialized training. Bachelor's degree programs in medical technology include courses in chemistry, biological sciences, microbiology, mathematics, statistics, and specialized courses devoted to knowledge and skills used in the clinical laboratory. Many programs also offer or require courses in management, business, and computer applications. The Clinical Laboratory Improvement Act (CLIA) requires technologists who perform certain highly complex tests to have at least an associate's degree. Medical and clinical laboratory technicians generally have either an associate's degree from a community or junior college or a certificate from a hospital, vocational or technical school, or from one of the U.S. Armed Forces. A few technicians learn their skills on the job. The National Accrediting Agency for Clinical Laboratory Sciences (NAACLS) fully accredits 503 programs for medical and clinical laboratory technologists, medical and clinical laboratory technicians, histologic technologists and technicians, and pathologists' assistants. NAACLS also approves 70 programs in phlebotomy, cytogenetic technology, molecular biology, and clinical assisting. Other nationally recognized accrediting agencies include the Commission on Accreditation of Allied Health Education Programs (CAAHEP) and the Accrediting Bureau of Health Education Schools (ABHES). Some States require laboratory personnel to be licensed or registered. Information on licensure is available from State departments of health or boards of occupational licensing. Certification is a voluntary process by which a nongovernmental organization, such as a professional society or certifying agency, grants recognition to an individual whose professional competence meets prescribed standards. Widely accepted by employers in the health industry, certification is a prerequisite for most jobs and often is necessary for advancement. Agencies certifying medical and clinical laboratory technologists and technicians include the Board of Registry of the American Society for Clinical Pathology, the American Medical Technologists, the National Credentialing Agency for Laboratory Personnel, and the Board of Registry of the American Association of Bioanalysts. These agencies have different requirements for certification and different organizational sponsors. Clinical laboratory personnel need good analytical judgment and the ability to work under pressure. Close attention to detail is essential, because small differences or changes in test substances or numerical readouts can be crucial for patient care. Manual dexterity and normal color vision are highly desirable. With the widespread use of automated laboratory equipment, computer skills are important. In addition, technologists in particular are expected to be good at problem solving.

Technologists may advance to supervisory positions in laboratory work or become chief medical or clinical laboratory technologists or laboratory managers in hospitals. Manufacturers of home diagnostic testing kits and laboratory equipment and supplies seek experienced technologists to work in product development, marketing, and sales. Graduate education in medical technology, one of the biological sciences, chemistry, management, or education usually speeds advancement. A doctorate is needed to become a laboratory director. However, federal regulation allows directors of moderate complexity laboratories to have either a master's degree or a bachelor's degree combined with the appropriate amount of training and experience. Technicians can become technologists through additional education and experience.

JOB OUTLOOK

Employment of clinical laboratory workers is expected to grow about as fast as the average for all occupations through the year 2010, as the volume of laboratory tests increases with population growth and the development of new types of tests. Technological advances will continue to have two opposing effects on employment through 2010. New, increasingly powerful diagnostic tests will encourage additional testing and spur employment. On the other hand, research and development efforts targeted at simplifying routine testing procedures may enhance the ability of nonlaboratory personnel, physicians and patients, in particular, to perform tests now done in laboratories. Although significant, growth will not be the only source of opportunities. As in most occupations, many openings will result from the need to replace workers who transfer to other occupations, retire, or stop working for some other reason.

EARNINGS

Median annual earnings of medical and clinical laboratory technologists were $40,510 in 2000. The middle 50 percent earned between $34,220 and $47,460. The lowest 10 percent earned less than $29,240, and the highest 10 percent earned more than $55,560. Median annual earnings in the industries employing the largest numbers of medical and clinical laboratory technologists in 2000 were as follows:

- Hospitals $40,840
- Medical and dental laboratories $39,780
- Offices and clinics of medical doctors $38,850

Median annual earnings of medical and clinical laboratory technicians were $27,540 in 2000. The middle 50 percent earned between $22,260 and $34,320. The lowest 10 percent earned less than $18,550, and the highest 10 percent earned more than $42,370.

Median annual earnings in the industries employing the largest numbers of medical and clinical laboratory technicians in 2000 were as follows:

- Hospitals $28,860
- Colleges and universities $27,810
- Offices and clinics of medical doctors $27,180
- Medical and dental laboratories $25,250
- Health and allied health services, not elsewhere classified $24,370

According to the American Society for Clinical Pathology, median hourly pay of staff clinical laboratory technologists and technicians in 2000 varied by specialty as follows:

	Beginning	Average	Top
Cytotechnologist	$16.70	$21.30	$24.00
Histotechnologist	$13.90	$18.00	$19.90
Medical technologist	$14.00	$17.90	$20.50
Histologic technician	$12.00	$15.30	$17.30
Medical laboratory technician	$11.40	$14.00	$16.30
Phlebotomist	$8.10	$9.90	$11.80

RELATED OCCUPATIONS

Clinical laboratory technologists and technicians analyze body fluids, tissue, and other substances using a variety of tests. Similar or related procedures are performed by chemists and material scientists, science technicians, and veterinary technologists, technicians, and assistants.

SOURCES OF ADDITIONAL INFORMATION

For a list of accredited and approved educational programs for clinical laboratory personnel, contact: National Accrediting Agency for Clinical Laboratory Sciences, 8410 W. Bryn Mawr Ave., Suite 670, Chicago, IL 60631. Internet: http://www.naacls.org

Information on certification is available from:

- American Association of Bioanalysts, 917 Locust St., Suite 1100, St. Louis, MO 63101. Internet: http://www.aab.org
- American Medical Technologists, 710 Higgins Rd., Park Ridge, IL 60068. Internet: http://www.amt1.com
- American Society for Clinical Pathology, Board of Registry, 2100 West Harrison St., Chicago, IL 60612. Internet: http://www.ascp.org/bor
- National Credentialing Agency for Laboratory Personnel, P.O. Box 15945-289, Lenexa, KS 66285-5935. Internet: http://www.nca-info.org

Additional career information is available from:

- American Association of Blood Banks, 8101 Glenbrook Rd., Bethesda, MD 20814-2749. Internet: http://www.aabb.org
- American Society for Clinical Laboratory Science, 7910 Woodmont Ave., Suite 530, Bethesda, MD 20814. Internet: http://www.ascls.org
- American Society for Clinical Pathology, 2100 West Harrison St., Chicago, IL 60612. Internet: http://www.ascp.org

Chapter 18

DENTAL HYGIENISTS

SIGNIFICANT POINTS

- Dental hygienists are projected to be one of the 30 fastest growing occupations.
- Population growth and greater retention of natural teeth will stimulate demand for dental hygienists.
- Opportunities for part-time work and flexible schedules are common.

NATURE OF THE WORK

Dental hygienists remove soft and hard deposits from teeth, teach patients how to practice good oral hygiene, and provide other preventive dental care. Hygienists examine patients' teeth and gums, recording the presence of diseases or abnormalities. They remove calculus, stains, and plaque from teeth; take and develop dental x rays; and apply cavity-preventive agents such as fluorides and pit and fissure sealants.

In some States, hygienists administer anesthetics; place and carve filling materials, temporary fillings, and periodontal dressings; remove sutures; perform root-planing as a periodontal therapy; and smooth and polish metal restorations. Although hygienists may not diagnose diseases, they can prepare clinical and laboratory diagnostic tests for the dentist to interpret. Hygienists sometimes work chairside with the dentist during treatment. Dental hygienists also help patients develop and maintain good oral health.

For example, they may explain the relationship between diet and oral health, or even the link between oral health and such serious conditions as heart disease and stroke. They also inform patients how to select toothbrushes and show them how to brush and floss their teeth. Dental hygienists use hand and rotary instruments and ultrasonics to clean and polish teeth, x-ray machines to take dental pictures, syringes with needles to administer local anesthetics, and models of teeth to explain oral hygiene.

Working Conditions

Flexible scheduling is a distinctive feature of this job. Full-time, part-time, evening, and weekend schedules are widely available. Dentists frequently hire hygienists to work only 2 or 3 days a week, so hygienists may hold jobs in more than one dental office. Dental hygienists work in clean, well-lighted offices. Important health safeguards include strict adherence to proper radiological procedures, and use of appropriate protective devices when administering anesthetic gas. Dental hygienists also wear safety glasses, surgical masks, and gloves to protect themselves from infectious diseases.

Employment

Dental hygienists held about 147,000 jobs in 2000. Because multiple jobholding is common in this field, the number of jobs exceeds the number of hygienists. More than half of all dental hygienists worked part time-less than 35 hours a week. Almost all dental hygienists work in private dental offices. Some work in public health agencies, hospitals, and clinics.

Training, Other Qualifications and Advancement

Dental hygienists must be licensed by the State in which they practice. To qualify for licensure, a candidate must graduate from an accredited dental hygiene school and pass both a written and clinical examination. The American Dental Association Joint Commission on National Dental

Examinations administers the written examination accepted by all States and the District of Columbia. State or regional testing agencies administer the clinical examination. In addition, most States require an examination on legal aspects of dental hygiene practice. Alabama allows candidates to take its examinations if they have been trained through a State-regulated on-the-job program in a dentist's office. In 2000, the Commission on Dental Accreditation accredited about 256 programs in dental hygiene. Although some programs lead to a bachelor's degree, most grant an associate degree. A dozen universities offer master's degree programs in dental hygiene or a related area. An associate degree is sufficient for practice in a private dental office. A bachelor's or master's degree usually is required for research, teaching, or clinical practice in public or school health programs. About half of the dental hygiene programs prefer applicants who have completed at least 1 year of college. However, requirements vary from one school to another. Schools offer laboratory, clinical, and classroom instruction in subjects such as anatomy, physiology, chemistry, microbiology, pharmacology, nutrition, radiography, histology (the study of tissue structure), periodontology (the study of gum diseases), pathology, dental materials, clinical dental hygiene, and social and behavioral sciences.

Dental hygienists should work well with others and must have good manual dexterity because they use dental instruments within a patient's mouth, with little room for error. High school students interested in becoming a dental hygienist should take courses in biology, chemistry, and mathematics.

JOB OUTLOOK

Employment of dental hygienists is expected to grow much faster than the average for all occupations through 2010, in response to increasing demand for dental care and the greater substitution of the services of hygienists for those previously performed by dentists. Job prospects are expected to remain very good unless the number of dental hygienist program graduates grows much faster than during the last decade, and results in a much larger pool of qualified applicants. Population growth and greater retention of natural teeth will stimulate demand for dental hygienists. Older dentists, who are less likely to employ dental hygienists, will leave and be replaced by recent graduates, who are more likely to do so. In addition, as dentists' workloads increase, they are expected to hire more hygienists to perform preventive dental care such as cleaning, so that they may devote their own time to more profitable procedures.

EARNINGS

Median hourly earnings of dental hygienists were $24.68 in 2000. The middle 50 percent earned between $20.46 and $29.72 an hour. The lowest 10 percent earned less than $15.53, and the highest 10 percent earned more than $35.39 an hour. Earnings vary by geographic location, employment setting, and years of experience.

Dental hygienists who work in private dental offices may be paid on an hourly, daily, salary, or commission basis. Benefits vary substantially by practice setting, and may be contingent upon full-time employment. According to the American Dental Association's 1999 Workforce Needs Assessment Survey, almost all full-time dental hygienists employed by private practitioners received paid vacation. The survey also found that 9 out of 10 full- and part-time dental hygienists received dental coverage. Dental hygienists who work for school systems, public health agencies, the Federal Government, or State agencies usually have substantial benefits.

RELATED OCCUPATIONS

Workers in other occupations supporting health practitioners in an office setting include dental assistants, medical assistants, occupational therapist assistants and aides, physical therapist assistants and aides, physician assistants, and registered nurses.

SOURCES OF ADDITIONAL INFORMATION

For information on a career in dental hygiene and the educational requirements to enter this occupation, contact: Division of Professional Development, American Dental Hygienists' Association, 444 N. Michigan Ave., Suite 3400, Chicago, IL 60611. Internet: http://www.adha.org

For information about accredited programs and educational requirements, contact: Commission on Dental Accreditation, American

Dental Association, 211 E. Chicago Ave., Suite 1814, Chicago, IL 60611. Internet: http://www.ada.org

The State Board of Dental Examiners in each State can supply information on licensing requirements.

Chapter 19

DIAGNOSTIC MEDICAL SONOGRAPHERS

SIGNIFICANT POINTS

- Sonographers should experience favorable job opportunities as ultrasound becomes an increasingly attractive alternative to radiologic procedures.
- More than half of all sonographers are employed by hospitals, and most of the remainder work in physicians' offices and clinics, including diagnostic imaging centers.
- Beginning in 2005, an associate or higher degree from an accredited program will be required for registration.

NATURE OF THE WORK

Diagnostic imaging embraces several procedures that aid in diagnosing ailments, the most familiar being the x ray. Another increasingly common diagnostic imaging method, called magnetic resonance imaging (MRI), uses giant magnets and radio waves rather than radiation to create an image. Not all imaging technologies use ionizing radiation or radio waves, however.

Sonography, or ultrasonography, is the use of sound waves to generate an image used for assessment and diagnosis of various medical conditions. Many people associate sonography with obstetrics and the viewing of the fetus in the womb. But this technology has many other applications in the diagnosis and treatment of medical conditions. Diagnostic medical sonographers, also known as ultrasonographers, use special equipment to direct nonionizing, high frequency sound waves into areas of the patient's body.

Sonographers operate the equipment, which collects reflected echoes and forms an image that may be videotaped, transmitted, or photographed for interpretation and diagnosis by a physician. Sonographers begin by explaining the procedure to the patient and recording any additional medical history that may be relevant to the condition being viewed. They then select appropriate equipment settings and direct the patient to move into positions that will provide the best view. To perform the exam, sonographers use a transducer, which transmits sound waves in a cone- or rectangle-shaped beam. Although techniques vary based on the area being examined, sonographers usually spread a special gel on the skin to aid the transmission of sound waves. Viewing the screen during the scan, sonographers look for subtle visual cues that contrast healthy areas from unhealthy ones. They decide whether the images are satisfactory for diagnostic purposes and select which ones to show to the physician. Diagnostic medical sonographers may specialize in obstetric and gynecologic sonography (the female reproductive system), abdominal sonography (the liver, kidneys, gallbladder, spleen, and pancreas), neurosonography (the brain), or ophthalmologic sonography (the eyes). In addition, sonographers also may specialize in vascular technology or echocardiography.

Obstetric and gynecologic sonographers specialize in the study of the female reproductive system. This includes one of the more well known uses of sonography: examining the fetus of a pregnant woman to track its growth and health.

Abdominal sonographers inspect a patient's abdominal cavity to help diagnose and treat conditions involving primarily the gallbladder, bile ducts, kidneys, liver, pancreas, and spleen. Abdominal sonographers also are able to scan parts of the heart, although diagnosis of the heart using ultrasound usually is done by echocardiographers.

Neurosonographers use ultrasound technology to focus on the nervous system, including the brain. In neonatal care, neurosonographers study and diagnose neurological and nervous system disorders in premature infants. They also may scan blood vessels to check for abnormalities indicating a stroke in infants diagnosed with sickle cell anemia. Like other sonographers, neurosonographers operate transducers to perform the ultrasound, but use different frequencies and beam shapes than obstetric and abdominal sonographers.

Ophthalmologic sonographers use ultrasound to study the eyes. Ultrasound aids in the insertion of prosthetic lenses by allowing accurate measurement of the eyes. Ophthalmologic ultrasound also helps diagnose and track tumors, blood supply conditions, separated retinas, and other ailments of the eye and the surrounding tissue. Ophthalmologic sonographers use high frequency transducers made exclusively to study the eyes, which are much smaller than those used in other specialties.

In addition to working directly with patients, diagnostic medical sonographers keep patient records and adjust and maintain equipment. They also may prepare work schedules, evaluate equipment purchases, or manage a sonography or diagnostic imaging department.

WORKING CONDITIONS

Most full-time sonographers work about 40 hours a week; they may have evening weekend hours and times when they are on call and must be ready to report to work on short notice. Sonographers typically work in healthcare facilities that are clean and well lit. Some travel to patients in large vans equipped with sophisticated diagnostic equipment. Sonographers are on their feet for long periods and may have to lift or turn disabled patients. They work at diagnostic imaging machines but may also do some procedures at patients' bedsides.

EMPLOYMENT

Diagnostic medical sonographers held about 33,000 jobs in 2000. More than half of all sonographer jobs are in hospitals. Most of the rest are in physicians' offices and clinics, primarily in offices specializing in obstetrics and in diagnostic imaging centers. According to the 2000 Sonography Benchmark Survey conducted by the Society of Diagnostic Medical Sonographers (SDMS), about three out of four sonographers worked in urban areas.

TRAINING, OTHER QUALIFICATIONS AND ADVANCEMENT

There are several avenues for entry into the field of diagnostic medical sonography. Sonographers may train in hospitals, vocational-technical institutions, colleges and universities, and the Armed Forces. Some training programs prefer applicants with a background in science or experience in other health professions, but also will consider high school graduates with courses in math and science, as well as applicants with liberal arts backgrounds.

Colleges and universities offer formal training in both 2- and 4-year programs, culminating in an associate or bachelor's degree. Two-year programs are most prevalent. Course work includes classes in anatomy, physiology, instrumentation, basic physics, patient care, and medical ethics.

The Joint Review Committee on Education for Diagnostic Medical Sonography accredits most formal training programs-76 programs in 1999. Some health workers, such as obstetric nurses and radiologic technologists, seek to increase their marketability by cross-training in fields such as sonography. Many take 1-year programs resulting in a certificate. Additionally, sonographers specializing in one discipline often seek competency in others; for example, obstetric sonographers might seek training in and exposure to abdominal sonography to broaden their opportunities.

While no State requires licensure in diagnostic medical sonography, the American Registry of Diagnostic Medical Sonographers (ARDMS) certifies the competency of sonographers through registration. Because registration provides an independent, objective measure of an individual's professional standing, many employers prefer to hire registered sonographers. Registration with ARDMS requires passing a general physics and instrumentation examination, in addition to passing an exam in a specialty such as obstetrics/gynecology, abdominal, or neurosonography.

While formal education is not necessary to take the exams, an associate or bachelor's degree from an accredited program is preferred. Beginning in 2005, ARDMS will consider for registration only those holding an associate or higher degree. To keep their registration current, sonographers must complete 30 hours of continuing education every 3 years to stay abreast of advances in the occupation and in technology.

Sonographers need good communication and interpersonal skills because they must be able to explain technical procedures and results to their patients, some of whom may be nervous about the exam or the problems it may reveal. They also should have some background in math and science, especially when they must perform mathematical and scientific calculations in analyses for diagnosis.

JOB OUTLOOK

Employment of diagnostic medical sonographers is expected to grow faster than the average for all occupations through 2010 as the population grows and ages, increasing the demand for diagnostic imaging and therapeutic technology. Some job openings also will arise from the need to replace sonographers who leave the occupation. Ultrasound is becoming an increasingly attractive alternative to radiologic procedures as patients seek safer treatment methods. Because ultrasound-unlike most diagnostic imaging methods-does not involve radiation, harmful side effects and complications from repeated use are rarer for both the patient and the sonographer.

Sonographic technology is expected to evolve rapidly and to spawn many new ultrasound procedures, such as 3D-ultrasonography for use in obstetric and ophthalmologic diagnosis. However, high costs may limit the rate at which some promising new technologies are adopted. Hospitals will remain the principal employer of diagnostic medical sonographers.

However, employment is expected to grow more rapidly in offices and clinics of physicians, including diagnostic imaging centers. Health facilities such as these are expected to grow very rapidly through 2010 due to the strong shift toward outpatient care, encouraged by third-party payers and made possible by technological advances that permit more procedures to be performed outside the hospital.

EARNINGS

Median annual earnings of diagnostic medical sonographers were $44,820 in 2000. The middle 50 percent earned between $38,390 and $52,750 a year. The lowest 10 percent earned less than $32,470, and the highest 10 percent earned more than $59,310. Median annual earnings of diagnostic medical sonographers in 2000 were $43,950 in hospitals and $46,190 in offices and clinics of medical doctors.

RELATED OCCUPATIONS

Diagnostic medical sonographers operate sophisticated equipment to help physicians and other health practitioners diagnose and treat patients. Workers in related occupations include cardiovascular technologists and technicians, clinical laboratory technologists and technicians, nuclear medicine technologists, radiologic technologists and technicians, and respiratory therapists.

SOURCES OF ADDITIONAL INFORMATION

For more information on a career as a diagnostic medical sonographer, contact:

- Society of Diagnostic Medical Sonographers, 2745 N. Dallas Parkway, Suite 350, Plano, TX 75093-8729. Internet: http://www.sdms.org
- The American Registry of Diagnostic Medical Sonographers, 600 Jefferson Plaza, Suite 360, Rockville, MD 20852-1150. Internet: http://www.ardms.org

For a current list of accredited education programs in diagnostic medical sonography, write to: The Joint Review Committee on Education in Diagnostic Medical Sonography, 1248 Harwood Rd., Bedford, TX 76021-4244. Internet: http://www.caahep.org

Chapter 20

EMERGENCY MEDICAL TECHNICIANS AND PARAMEDICS

SIGNIFICANT POINTS

- Job stress is common due to irregular hours and treating patients in life-or-death situations.
- Formal training and certification are required but State requirements vary.
- Employment is projected to grow faster than average as paid emergency medical technician positions replace unpaid volunteers.

NATURE OF THE WORK

People's lives often depend on the quick reaction and competent care of emergency medical technicians (EMTs) and paramedics, EMTs with additional advanced training to perform more difficult pre-hospital medical procedures. Incidents as varied as automobile accidents, heart attacks, drownings, childbirth, and gunshot wounds all require immediate medical attention. EMTs and paramedics provide this vital attention as they care for and transport the sick or injured to a medical facility.

Depending on the nature of the emergency, EMTs and paramedics typically are dispatched to the scene by a 911 operator and often work with police and fire department personnel. Once they arrive, they determine the nature and extent of the patient's condition while trying to ascertain whether the patient has preexisting medical problems. Following strict rules and guidelines, they give appropriate emergency care and, when necessary, transport the patient.

Some paramedics are trained to treat patients with minor injuries on the scene of an accident or at their home without transporting them to a medical facility. Emergency treatments for more complicated problems are carried out under the direction of medical doctors by radio preceding or during transport. EMTs and paramedics may use special equipment such as backboards to immobilize patients before placing them on stretchers and securing them in the ambulance for transport to a medical facility. Usually, one EMT or paramedic drives while the other monitors the patient's vital signs and gives additional care as needed. Some EMTs work as part of the flight crew of helicopters that transport critically ill or injured patients to hospital trauma centers.

At the medical facility, EMTs and paramedics help transfer patients to the emergency department, report their observations and actions to staff, and may provide additional emergency treatment. After each run, EMTs and paramedics replace used supplies and check equipment. If a transported patient had a contagious disease, EMTs and paramedics decontaminate the interior of the ambulance and report cases to the proper authorities.

Beyond these general duties, the specific responsibilities of EMTs and paramedics depend on their level of qualification and training. To determine this, the National Registry of Emergency Medical Technicians (NREMT) registers emergency medical service (EMS) providers at four levels: First Responder, EMT-Basic, EMT-Intermediate, and EMT-Paramedic. Some States, however, do their own certification and use numeric ratings from 1 to 4 to distinguish levels of proficiency.

The lowest level-First Responders-are trained to provide basic emergency medical care because they tend to be the first persons to arrive at the scene of an incident. Many firefighters, police officers, and other emergency workers have this level of training. The EMT-Basic, also known as EMT-1, represents the first component of the emergency medical technician system. An EMT-1 is trained to care for patients on accident scenes and on transport by ambulance to the hospital under medical direction. The EMT-1 has the emergency skills to assess a patient's condition and manage respiratory, cardiac, and trauma emergencies.

The EMT-Intermediate (EMT-2 and EMT-3) has more advanced training that allows administration of intravenous fluids, use of manual defibrillators to give lifesaving shocks to a stopped heart, and use of advanced airway techniques and equipment to assist patients experiencing respiratory emergencies.

EMT-Paramedics (EMT-4) provide the most extensive pre-hospital care. In addition to the procedures already described, paramedics may administer drugs orally and intravenously, interpret electrocardiograms (EKGs), perform endotracheal intubations, and use monitors and other complex equipment.

WORKING CONDITIONS

EMTs and paramedics work both indoors and outdoors, in all types of weather. They are required to do considerable kneeling, bending, and heavy lifting. These workers risk noise-induced hearing loss from sirens and back injuries from lifting patients. In addition, EMTs and paramedics may be exposed to diseases such as Hepatitis-B and AIDS, as well as violence from drug overdose victims or mentally unstable patients. The work is not only physically strenuous, but also stressful, involving life-or-death situations and suffering patients. Nonetheless, many people find the work exciting and challenging and enjoy the opportunity to help others. EMTs and paramedics employed by fire departments work about 50 hours a week. Those employed by hospitals frequently work between 45 and 60 hours a week, and those in private ambulance services, between 45 and 50 hours. Some of these workers, especially those in police and fire departments, are on call for extended periods. Because emergency services function 24 hours a day, EMTs and paramedics have irregular working hours that add to job stress.

EMPLOYMENT

EMTs and paramedics held about 172,000 jobs in 2000. Most career EMTs and paramedics work in metropolitan areas. There are many more volunteer EMTs and paramedics, especially in smaller cities, towns, and rural areas. They volunteer for fire departments, emergency medical services (EMS), or hospitals and may respond to only a few calls for service per month, or may answer the majority of calls, especially in smaller communities.

EMTs and paramedics work closely with firefighters, who often are certified as EMTs as well and act as first responders. Full- and part-time paid

EMTs and paramedics were employed in a number of industries. About 4 out of 10 worked in local and suburban transportation, as employees of private ambulance services. About 3 out of 10 worked in local government for fire departments, public ambulance services and EMS. Another 2 out 10 were found in hospitals, where they worked full time within the medical facility or responded to calls in ambulances or helicopters to transport critically ill or injured patients. The remainder worked in various industries providing emergency services.

TRAINING, OTHER QUALIFICATIONS AND ADVANCEMENT

Formal training and certification is needed to become an EMT or paramedic. All 50 States possess a certification procedure. In 38 States and the District of Columbia, registration with the National Registry of Emergency Medical Technicians (NREMT) is required at some or all levels of certification. Other States administer their own certification examination or provide the option of taking the NREMT examination.

To maintain certification, EMTs and paramedics must reregister, usually every 2 years. In order to re-register, an individual must be working as an EMT or paramedic and meet a continuing education requirement. Training is offered at progressive levels: EMT-Basic, also known as EMT-1; EMT-Intermediate, or EMT-2 and EMT-3; and EMT-paramedic, or EMT-4. The EMT-Basic represents the first level of skills required to work in the emergency medical system.

Coursework typically emphasizes emergency skills such as managing respiratory, trauma, and cardiac emergencies and patient assessment. Formal courses are often combined with time in an emergency room or ambulance. The program also provides instruction and practice in dealing with bleeding, fractures, airway obstruction, cardiac arrest, and emergency childbirth. Students learn to use and maintain common emergency equipment, such as backboards, suction devices, splints, oxygen delivery systems, and stretchers.

Graduates of approved EMT basic training programs who pass a written and practical examination administered by the State certifying agency or the NREMT earn the title of Registered EMT-Basic. The course also is a prerequisite for EMT-Intermediate and EMT-Paramedic training. EMT-Intermediate training requirements vary from State to State. Applicants can opt to receive training in EMT-Shock Trauma, where the caregiver learns to start intravenous fluids and give certain medications, or in EMT-Cardiac, which includes learning heart rhythms and administering advanced medications. Training commonly includes 35 to 55 hours of additional instruction beyond EMT-Basic coursework and covers patient assessment, as well as the use of advanced airway devices and intravenous fluids.

Prerequisites for taking the EMT-Intermediate examination include registration as an EMT-Basic, required classroom work, and a specified amount of clinical experience. The most advanced level of training for this occupation is EMT-Paramedic. At this level, the caregiver receives additional training in body function and more advanced skills. The Paramedic Technology program usually lasts up to 2 years and results in an associate degree in applied science. Such education prepares the graduate to take the NREMT examination and become certified as an EMT-Paramedic. Extensive related coursework and clinical and field experience is required. Due to the longer training requirement, almost all EMT-Paramedics are in paid positions. Refresher courses and continuing education are available for EMTs and paramedics at all levels.

EMTs and paramedics should be emotionally stable, have good dexterity, agility, and physical coordination, and be able to lift and carry heavy loads. They also need good eyesight (corrective lenses may be used) with accurate color vision. Advancement beyond the EMT-Paramedic level usually means leaving fieldwork. An EMT-Paramedic can become a supervisor, operations manager, administrative director, or executive director of emergency services. Some EMTs and paramedics become instructors, dispatchers, or physician assistants, while others move into sales or marketing of emergency medical equipment. A number of people become EMTs and paramedics to assess their interest in healthcare and then decide to return to school and become registered nurses, physicians, or other health workers.

JOB OUTLOOK

Employment of emergency medical technicians and paramedics is expected to grow faster than the average for all occupations through 2010. Population growth and urbanization will increase the demand for full-time paid EMTs and paramedics rather than for volunteers. In addition, a large segment of the population-the aging baby boomers-will further spur demand for EMT services, as they become more likely to have medical emergencies.

There will still be demand for part-time, volunteer EMTs and paramedics in rural areas and smaller metropolitan areas. In addition to job growth, openings will occur because of replacement needs; some workers leave because of stressful working conditions, limited advancement potential, and the modest pay and benefits in the private sector. Most opportunities for EMTs and paramedics are expected to arise in hospitals and private ambulance services. Competition will be greater for jobs in local government, including fire, police, and independent third service rescue squad departments, where salaries and benefits tend to be slightly better. Opportunities will be best for those who have advanced certifications, such as EMT-Intermediate and EMT-Paramedic, as clients and patients demand higher levels of care before arriving at the hospital.

EARNINGS

Earnings of EMTs and paramedics depend on the employment setting and geographic location as well as the individual's training and experience. Median annual earnings of EMTs and paramedics were $22,460 in 2000. The middle 50 percent earned between $17,930 and $29,270. The lowest 10 percent earned less than $14,660, and the highest 10 percent earned more than $37,760. Median annual earnings in the industries employing the largest numbers of EMTs and paramedics in 2000 were:

- Local government $24,800
- Hospitals $23,590
- Local and suburban transportation $20,950

Those in emergency medical services who are part of fire or police departments receive the same benefits as firefighters or police officers. For example, many are covered by pension plans that provide retirement at half pay after 20 or 25 years of service or if disabled in the line of duty.

RELATED OCCUPATIONS

Other workers in occupations that require quick and level-headed reactions to life-or-death situations are air traffic controllers, firefighting occupations, physician assistants, police and detectives, and registered nurses.

SOURCES OF ADDITIONAL INFORMATION

General information about emergency medical technicians and paramedics is available from:

- National Association of Emergency Medical Technicians, 408 Monroe St., Clinton, MS 39056. Internet: http://www.naemt.org
- National Registry of Emergency Medical Technicians, P.O. Box 29233, Columbus, OH 43229. Internet: http://www.nremt.org
- National Highway Transportation Safety Administration, EMS Division, 400 7th St. SW., NTS-14, Washington, DC. Internet: http://www.nhtsa.dot.gov/people/injury/ems

Chapter 21

LICENSED PRACTICAL AND LICENSED VOCATIONAL NURSES

SIGNIFICANT POINTS

- Training lasting about 1 year is available in about 1,100 State-approved programs, mostly in vocational or technical schools.
- Nursing homes will offer the most new jobs.
- Job seekers in hospitals may face competition as the number of hospital jobs for LPNs declines.

NATURE OF THE WORK

Licensed practical nurses (LPNs), or licensed vocational nurses (LVNs) as they are called in Texas and California, care for the sick, injured, convalescent, and disabled under the direction of physicians and registered nurses. Most LPNs provide basic bedside care. They take vital signs such as temperature, blood pressure, pulse, and respiration. They also treat bedsores, prepare and give injections and enemas, apply dressings, give alcohol rubs and massages, apply ice packs and hot water bottles, and monitor catheters. LPNs observe patients and report adverse reactions to medications or treatments. They collect samples for testing, perform routine laboratory tests, feed patients, and record food and fluid intake and output. They help patients with bathing, dressing, and personal hygiene, keep them comfortable, and care for their emotional needs. In States where the law allows, they may administer prescribed medicines or start intravenous fluids. Some LPNs help deliver, care for, and feed infants.

Experienced LPNs may supervise nursing assistants and aides. LPNs in nursing homes provide routine bedside care, help evaluate residents' needs, develop care plans, and supervise the care provided by nursing aides. In doctors' offices and clinics, they also may make appointments, keep records, and perform other clerical duties. LPNs who work in private homes also may prepare meals and teach family members simple nursing tasks.

WORKING CONDITIONS

Most licensed practical nurses in hospitals and nursing homes work a 40-hour week, but because patients need around-the-clock care, some work nights, weekends, and holidays. They often stand for long periods and help patients move in bed, stand, or walk. LPNs may face hazards from caustic chemicals, radiation, and infectious diseases such as hepatitis. They are subject to back injuries when moving patients and shock from electrical equipment. They often must deal with the stress of heavy workloads. In addition, the patients they care for may be confused, irrational, agitated, or uncooperative.

EMPLOYMENT

Licensed practical nurses held about 700,000 jobs in 2000. Twenty-nine percent of LPNs worked in nursing homes, 28 percent worked in hospitals, and 14 percent in physicians' offices and clinics. Others worked for home healthcare services, residential care facilities, schools, temporary help agencies, or government agencies; about 1 in 5 worked part time.

TRAINING, OTHER QUALIFICATIONS AND ADVANCEMENT

All States and the District of Columbia require LPNs to pass a licensing examination after completing a State- approved practical nursing program. A high school diploma, or equivalent, usually is required for entry, although some programs accept candidates without a diploma or are designed as part of a high school curriculum.

In 2000, approximately 1,100 State-approved programs provided practical nursing training. Almost 6 out of 10 students were enrolled in technical or vocational schools, while 3 out of 10 were in community and junior colleges. Others were in high schools, hospitals, and colleges and universities. Most practical nursing programs last about 1 year and include both classroom study and supervised clinical practice (patient care). Classroom study covers basic nursing concepts and patient-care related subjects, including anatomy, physiology, medical-surgical nursing, pediatrics, obstetrics, psychiatric nursing, administration of drugs, nutrition, and first aid. Clinical practice usually is in a hospital, but sometimes includes other settings.

LPNs should have a caring, sympathetic nature. They should be emotionally stable because work with the sick and injured can be stressful. They also should have keen observational, decision making, and communication skills. As part of a healthcare team, they must be able to follow orders and work under close supervision.

JOB OUTLOOK

Employment of LPNs is expected to grow about as fast as the average for all occupations through 2010 in response to the long-term care needs of a rapidly growing elderly population and the general growth of healthcare. Replacement needs will be a major source of job openings, as many workers leave the occupation permanently.

Employment of LPNs in nursing homes is expected to grow faster than the average. Nursing homes will offer the most new jobs for LPNs as the number of aged and disabled persons in need of long-term care rises. In addition to caring for the aged and disabled, nursing homes will be called on to care for the increasing number of patients who have been discharged from the hospital but who have not recovered enough to return home.

LPNs seeking positions in hospitals may face competition, as the number of hospital jobs for LPNs declines. An increasing proportion of sophisticated procedures, which once were performed only in hospitals, are being performed in physicians' offices and clinics, including ambulatory surgicenters and emergency medical centers, due largely to advances in technology. As a result, employment of LPNs is projected to grow much faster than average in these places as healthcare expands outside the traditional hospital setting.

Employment of LPNs is expected to grow much faster than average in home healthcare services. This is in response to a growing number of older persons with functional disabilities, consumer preference for care in the home, and technological advances, which make it possible to bring increasingly complex treatments into the home.

EARNINGS

Median annual earnings of licensed practical nurses were $29,440 in 2000. The middle 50 percent earned between $24,920 and $34,800. The lowest 10 percent earned less than $21,520, and the highest 10 percent earned more than $41,800. Median annual earnings in the industries employing the largest numbers of licensed practical nurses in 2000 were as follows:

- Personnel supply services $35,750
- Home health care services $31,220
- Nursing and personal care facilities $29,980
- Hospitals $28,450
- Offices and clinics of medical doctors $27,520

RELATED OCCUPATIONS

LPNs work closely with people while helping them. So do emergency medical technicians and paramedics, social and human service assistants, surgical technologists, and teacher assistants.

SOURCES OF ADDITIONAL INFORMATION

For information about practical nursing, contact:

- National League for Nursing, 61 Broadway, New York, NY 10006. Internet: http://www.nln.org

- National Association for Practical Nurse Education and Service, Inc., 8607 Second Avenue, Suite 404-A, Silver Spring, MD 20910.
- National Federation of Licensed Practical Nurses, Inc., 893 US Highway 70 West, Suite 202, Garner, NC 27529-2597.

Chapter 22

MEDICAL RECORDS AND HEALTH INFORMATION TECHNICIANS

SIGNIFICANT POINTS

- Medical records and health information technicians are projected to be one of the fastest growing occupations.
- High school students can improve chances of acceptance into a medical record and health information education program by taking anatomy, physiology, medical terminology, and computer courses.
- Most technicians will be employed by hospitals, but job growth will be faster in offices and clinics of physicians, nursing homes, and home health agencies.

NATURE OF THE WORK

Every time health care personnel treat a patient, they record what they observed, and how the patient was treated medically. This record includes information the patient provides concerning their symptoms and medical history, the results of examinations, reports of x rays and laboratory tests, diagnoses, and treatment plans. Medical records and health information technicians organize and evaluate these records for completeness and accuracy. Medical records and health information technicians begin to assemble patients' health information by first making sure their initial medical charts are complete. They ensure all forms are completed and properly identified and signed, and all necessary information is in the computer. Sometimes, they communicate with physicians or others to clarify diagnoses or get additional information. Technicians assign a code to each diagnosis and procedure. They consult classification manuals and rely, also, on their knowledge of disease processes. Technicians then use a software program to assign the patient to one of several hundred "diagnosis-related groups," or DRGs. The DRG determines the amount the hospital will be reimbursed if the patient is covered by Medicare or other insurance programs using the DRG system.

Technicians who specialize in coding are called health information coders, medical record coders, coder/abstractors, or coding specialists. In addition to the DRG system, coders use other coding systems, such as those geared towards ambulatory settings. Technicians also use computer programs to tabulate and analyze data to help improve patient care, control costs, for use in legal actions, in response to surveys, or for use in research studies.

Tumor registrars compile and maintain records of patients who have cancer to provide information to physicians and for research studies. Medical records and health information technicians' duties vary with the size of the facility.

In large to medium facilities, technicians may specialize in one aspect of health information, or supervise health information clerks and transcriptionists while a medical records and health information administrator manages the department. In small facilities, a credentialed medical records and health information technician sometimes manages the department.

Working Conditions

Medical records and health information technicians usually work a 40-hour week. Some overtime may be required. In hospitals-where health information departments often are open 24 hours a day, 7 days a week-technicians may work day, evening, and night shifts. Medical records and health information technicians work in pleasant and comfortable offices. This is one of the few health occupations in which there is little or no physical contact with patients. Because accuracy is essential, technicians must pay close attention to detail. Technicians who work at computer monitors for prolonged periods must guard against eyestrain and muscle pain.

EMPLOYMENT

Medical records and health information technicians held about 136,000 jobs in 2000. About 4 out of 10 jobs were in hospitals. The rest were mostly in nursing homes, medical group practices, clinics, and home health agencies. Insurance firms that deal in health matters employ a small number of health information technicians to tabulate and analyze health information. Public health departments also hire technicians to supervise data collection from health care institutions and to assist in research.

TRAINING, OTHER QUALIFICATIONS AND ADVANCEMENT

Medical records and health information technicians entering the field usually have an associate degree from a community or junior college. In addition to general education, coursework includes medical terminology, anatomy and physiology, legal aspects of health information, coding and abstraction of data, statistics, database management, quality improvement methods, and computer training. Applicants can improve their chances of admission into a program by taking biology, chemistry, health, and computer courses in high school.

Hospitals sometimes advance promising health information clerks to jobs as medical records and health information technicians, although this practice may be less common in the future. Advancement usually requires 2 to 4 years of job experience and completion of a hospital's in-house training program.

Most employers prefer to hire Registered Health Information Technicians (RHIT), who must pass a written examination offered by AHIMA. To take the examination, a person must graduate from a 2-year associate degree program accredited by the Commission on Accreditation of Allied Health Education Programs (CAAHEP) of the American Medical Association. Technicians trained in non-CAAHEP accredited programs, or on the job, are not eligible to take the examination. In 2001, CAAHEP accredited 177 programs for health information technicians. Technicians who specialize in coding may also obtain voluntary certification.

Experienced medical records and health information technicians usually advance in one of two ways-by specializing or managing. Many senior technicians specialize in coding, particularly Medicare coding, or in tumor registry. In large medical records and health information departments, experienced technicians may advance to section supervisor, overseeing the work of the coding, correspondence, or discharge sections, for example. Senior technicians with RHIT credentials may become director or assistant director of a medical records and health information department in a small facility. However, in larger institutions, the director is usually an administrator, with a bachelor's degree in medical records and health information administration.

JOB OUTLOOK

Job prospects for formally trained technicians should be very good. Employment of medical records and health information technicians is expected to grow much faster than the average for all occupations through 2010, due to rapid growth in the number of medical tests, treatments, and procedures which will be increasingly scrutinized by third-party payers, regulators, courts, and consumers. Hospitals will continue to employ a large percentage of health information technicians, but growth will not be as fast as in other areas. Increasing demand for detailed records in offices and clinics of physicians should result in fast employment growth, especially in large group practices. Rapid growth is also expected in nursing homes and home health agencies.

EARNINGS

Median annual earnings of medical records and health information technicians were $22,750 in 2000. The middle 50 percent earned between $18,700 and $28,590. The lowest 10 percent earned less than $15,710, and the highest 10 percent earned more than $35,170. Median annual earnings in the industries employing the largest numbers of medical records and health information technicians in 2000 were as follows:

- Nursing and personal care facilities $23,760
- Hospitals $23,540
- Offices and clinics of medical doctors $21,090

RELATED OCCUPATIONS

Medical records and health information technicians need a strong clinical background to analyze the contents of medical records. Workers in other occupations requiring knowledge of medical terminology, anatomy, and physiology without physical contact with the patient are medical secretaries and medical transcriptionists.

SOURCES OF ADDITIONAL INFORMATION

Information on careers in medical records and health information technology, including a list of CAAHEP- accredited programs is available from: American Health Information Management Association, 233 N. Michigan Ave., Suite 2150, Chicago, IL 60601-5800. Internet: http://www.ahima.org

Chapter 23

NUCLEAR MEDICINE TECHNOLOGISTS

SIGNIFICANT POINTS

- Faster-than-average growth will arise from an increase in the number of middle-aged and elderly persons, who are the primary users of diagnostic procedures.
- Technologists with cross training in radiologic technology or other modalities will have the best prospects.

NATURE OF THE WORK

In nuclear medicine, radionuclides-unstable atoms that emit radiation spontaneously-are used to diagnose and treat disease. Radionuclides are purified and compounded like other drugs to form radiopharmaceuticals. Nuclear medicine technologists administer these radiopharmaceuticals to patients, then monitor the characteristics and functions of tissues or organs in which they localize. Abnormal areas show higher or lower concentrations of radioactivity than normal.

Nuclear medicine technologists operate cameras that detect and map the radioactive drug in the patient's body to create an image on photographic film or a computer monitor.

Radiologic technologists and technicians also operate diagnostic imaging equipment, but their equipment creates an image by projecting an x ray through the patient. Nuclear medicine technologists explain test procedures to patients. They prepare a dosage of the radiopharmaceutical and administer it by mouth, injection, or other means. When preparing radiopharmaceuticals, technologists adhere to safety standards that keep the radiation dose to workers and patients as low as possible. Technologists position patients and start a gamma scintillation camera, or "scanner," which creates images of the distribution of a radiopharmaceutical as it localizes in and emits signals from the patient's body. Technologists produce the images on a computer screen or on film for a physician to interpret.

Some nuclear medicine studies, such as cardiac function studies, are processed with the aid of a computer. Nuclear medicine technologists also perform radioimmunoassay studies that assess the behavior of a radioactive substance inside the body. For example, technologists may add radioactive substances to blood or serum to determine levels of hormones or therapeutic drug content. Technologists keep patient records and record the amount and type of radionuclides received, used, and disposed of.

Working Conditions

Nuclear medicine technologists generally work a 40-hour week. This may include evening or weekend hours in departments that operate on an extended schedule. Opportunities for part-time and shift work are also available. In addition, technologists in hospitals may have on-call duty on a rotational basis. Because technologists are on their feet much of the day, and may lift or turn disabled patients, physical stamina is important. Although there is potential for radiation exposure in this field, it is kept to a minimum by the use of shielded syringes, gloves, and other protective devices and adherence to strict radiation safety guidelines. Technologists also wear badges that measure radiation levels. Because of safety programs, however, badge measurements rarely exceed established safety levels.

Employment

Nuclear medicine technologists held about 18,000 jobs in 2000. About two-thirds of all jobs were in hospitals. The rest were in physicians' offices and clinics, including diagnostic imaging centers.

TRAINING, OTHER QUALIFICATIONS AND ADVANCEMENT

Nuclear medicine technology programs range in length from 1 to 4 years and lead to a certificate, associate's degree, or bachelor's degree. Generally, certificate programs are offered in hospitals, associate programs in community colleges, and bachelor's programs in 4-year colleges and in universities. Courses cover physical sciences, the biological effects of radiation exposure, radiation protection and procedures, the use of radiopharmaceuticals, imaging techniques, and computer applications. One-year certificate programs are for health professionals, especially radiologic technologists and diagnostic medical sonographers, who wish to specialize in nuclear medicine. They also attract medical technologists, registered nurses, and others who wish to change fields or specialize. Others interested in the nuclear medicine technology field have three options: A 2-year certificate program, a 2-year associate program, or a 4-year bachelor's program. The Joint Review Committee on Education Programs in Nuclear Medicine Technology accredits most formal training programs in nuclear medicine technology.

In 2000, there were 95 accredited programs in the continental United States and Puerto Rico. All nuclear medicine technologists must meet the minimum Federal standards on the administration of radioactive drugs and the operation of radiation detection equipment. In addition, about half of all States require technologists to be licensed. Technologists also may obtain voluntary professional certification or registration. Registration or certification is available from the American Registry of Radiologic Technologists and from the Nuclear Medicine Technology Certification Board.

Most employers prefer to hire certified or registered technologists. Nuclear medicine technologists should be sensitive to patients' physical and psychological needs. They must pay attention to detail, follow instructions, and work as part of a team. In addition, operating complicated equipment requires mechanical ability and manual dexterity.

Technologists may advance to supervisor, then to chief technologist, and to department administrator or director. Some technologists specialize in a clinical area such as nuclear cardiology or computer analysis or leave patient care to take positions in research laboratories. Some become instructors or directors in nuclear medicine technology programs, a step that usually requires a bachelor's degree or a master's in nuclear medicine technology.

Others leave the occupation to work as sales or training representatives for medical equipment and radiopharmaceutical manufacturing firms, or as radiation safety officers in regulatory agencies or hospitals.

JOB OUTLOOK

Employment of nuclear medicine technologists is expected to grow faster than the average for all occupations through the year 2010. The number of openings each year will be very low because the occupation is small. Growth will arise from an increase in the number of middle-aged and older persons who are the primary users of diagnostic procedures, including nuclear medicine tests. Technological innovations may increase the diagnostic uses of nuclear medicine. One example is the use of radiopharmaceuticals in combination with monoclonal antibodies to detect cancer at far earlier stages than is customary today, and without resorting to surgery. Another is the use of radionuclides to examine the heart's ability to pump blood. Wider use of nuclear medical imaging to observe metabolic and biochemical changes for neurology, cardiology, and oncology procedures, also will spur some demand for nuclear medicine technologists. On the other hand, cost considerations will affect the speed with which new applications of nuclear medicine grow. Some promising nuclear medicine procedures, such as positron emission tomography (PET), are extremely costly, and hospitals contemplating them will have to consider equipment costs, reimbursement policies, and the number of potential users.

EARNINGS

Median annual earnings of nuclear medicine technologists were $44,130 in 2000. The middle 50 percent earned between $38,150 and $52,190. The lowest 10 percent earned less than $31,910, and the highest 10 percent earned more than $58,500. Median annual earnings of nuclear medicine technologists in 2000 were $44,000 in hospitals.

RELATED OCCUPATIONS

Nuclear medical technologists operate sophisticated equipment to help physicians and other health practitioners diagnose and treat patients. Cardiovascular technologists and technicians, clinical laboratory technologists and technicians, diagnostic medical sonographers, radiation therapists, radiologic technologists and technicians, and respiratory therapists also perform similar functions.

SOURCES OF ADDITIONAL INFORMATION

Additional information on a career as a nuclear medicine technologist is available from: The Society of Nuclear Medicine-Technologist Section, 1850 Samuel Morse Dr., Reston, VA 22090. Internet: http://www.snm.org

For career information, send a stamped, self-addressed business size envelope with your request to: American Society of Radiologic Technologists, Customer Service Department, 15000 Central Ave. SE., Albuquerque, NM 87123-3917, or call (800) 444-2778. Internet: http://www.asrt.org/asrt.htm

For a list of accredited programs in nuclear medicine technology, write to: Joint Review Committee on Educational Programs in Nuclear Medicine Technology, PMB 418, 1 2nd Avenue East, Suite C, Polson, MT 59860-2107. Internet: http://www.jrcnmt.org

Information on certification is available from:

- American Registry of Radiologic Technologists, 1255 Northland Dr., St. Paul, MN 55120-1155. Internet: http://www.arrt.org
- Nuclear Medicine Technology Certification Board, 2970 Clairmont Rd., Suite 610, Atlanta, GA 30329. Internet: http://www.nmtcb.org

Chapter 24

OCCUPATIONAL HEALTH AND SAFETY SPECIALISTS AND TECHNICIANS

SIGNIFICANT POINTS

- Almost half of occupational health and safety specialists and technicians work in Federal, State, and local government agencies that enforce rules on health and safety.
- For positions as specialists, many employers, including the Federal Government, require 4-year college degrees in safety or a related field.

NATURE OF THE WORK

Occupational health and safety specialists and technicians, also known as occupational health and safety inspectors and industrial hygienists, help keep workplaces safe and workers unscathed. They promote occupational health and safety within organizations by developing safer, healthier, and more efficient ways of working.

Occupational health and safety specialists analyze work environments and design programs to control, eliminate, and prevent disease or injury caused by chemical, physical, and biological agents or ergonomic factors. They may conduct inspections and enforce adherence to laws, regulations, or employer policies governing worker health and safety. Occupational health and safety technicians collect data on work environments for analysis by occupational health and safety specialists. Usually working under the supervision of specialists, they help implement and evaluate programs designed to limit risks to workers. Occupational health and safety specialists and technicians identify hazardous conditions and practices.

Sometimes, they develop methods to predict hazards from experience, historical data, and other information sources. Then they identify potential hazards in existing or future systems, equipment, products, facilities, or processes. After reviewing the causes or effects of hazards, they evaluate the probability and severity of accidents that may result. For example, they might uncover patterns in injury data that implicate a specific cause such as system failure, human error, incomplete or faulty decision making, or a weakness in existing policies or practices. Then they develop and help enforce a plan to eliminate hazards, conducting training sessions for management, supervisors, and workers on health and safety practices and regulations, as necessary.

Lastly, they may check on the progress of the safety plan after its implementation. If improvements are not satisfactory, a new plan might be designed and put into practice.

Many occupational health and safety specialists inspect and test machinery and equipment, such as lifting devices, machine shields, or scaffolding, to ensure they meet appropriate safety regulations. They may check that personal protective equipment, such as masks, respirators, safety glasses, or safety helmets, is being used in workplaces according to regulations. They also check that dangerous materials are stored correctly. They test and identify work areas for potential accident and health hazards, such as toxic fumes and explosive gas-air mixtures, and may implement appropriate control measures, such as adjustments to ventilation systems. Their investigations might involve talking with workers and observing their work, as well as inspecting elements in their work environment, such as lighting, tools, and equipment. To measure and control hazardous substances, such as the noise or radiation levels, occupational health and safety specialists and technicians prepare and calibrate scientific equipment. Samples of dust, gases, vapors, and other potentially toxic materials must be collected and handled properly to ensure safety and accurate test results. If an accident occurs, occupational health and safety specialists help investigate unsafe working conditions, study possible causes, and recommend remedial action.

Some occupational health and safety specialists and technicians assist with the rehabilitation of workers after accidents and injuries, and make sure they return to work successfully. Frequent communication with management may be necessary to report on the status of occupational health and safety programs. Consultation with engineers or physicians also may be required. Occupational health and safety specialists prepare reports including observations, analysis of contaminants, and recommendation for control and correction of hazards. Those who develop expertise in certain areas may develop occupational health and safety systems, including policies, procedures, and manuals.

WORKING CONDITIONS

Occupational health and safety specialists and technicians work with many different people in a variety of environments. Their jobs often involve considerable fieldwork, and some travel frequently. Many occupational health and safety specialists and technicians work long and often irregular hours. Occupational health and safety specialists and technicians may experience unpleasant, stressful, and dangerous working conditions. For example, health and safety inspectors are exposed to many of the same physically strenuous conditions and hazards as industrial employees, and the work may be performed in unpleasant, stressful, and dangerous working conditions. Health and safety inspectors may find themselves in adversarial roles when the organization or individual being inspected objects to the process or its consequences.

EMPLOYMENT

Occupational health and safety specialists and technicians held about 35,000 jobs in 2000. The Federal Government-chiefly the Department of Labor-employed 8 percent, State governments employed 17 percent, and local governments employed 19 percent. The remainder were employed throughout the private sector in schools, hospitals, management consulting firms, public utilities, and manufacturing firms. Within the Federal government, most jobs are as Occupational Health and Safety Administration (OSHA) inspectors, who enforce U.S. Department of Labor regulations that ensure adequate safety principles, practices, and techniques are applied in workplaces. Employers may be fined for violation of OSHA standards. Within the U.S. Department of Health and Human Services, occupational health and safety specialists working for the National Institute of Occupational Safety and Health (NIOSH) provide private companies with an avenue to evaluate the health and safety of their employees without the risk of being fined. Most large government agencies also employ occupational health and safety specialists and technicians who work to protect agency employees. Most private companies either employ their own safety personnel or contract safety professionals to ensure OSHA compliance, as needed.

TRAINING, OTHER QUALIFICATIONS AND ADVANCEMENT

Requirements include a combination of education, experience, and passing scores on written examinations. Many employers, including the Federal Government, require a 4-year college degree in safety or a related field for some positions.

Experience as a safety professional is also a prerequisite for many positions. All occupational health and safety specialists and technicians are trained in the applicable laws or inspection procedures through some combination of classroom and on-the-job training. In general, people who want to enter this occupation should be responsible and like detailed work. Occupational health and safety specialists and technicians should be able to communicate well. Recommended high school courses include English, chemistry, biology, and physics.

Certification is available through the Board of Certified Safety Professionals (BCSP) and the American Board of Industrial Hygiene (ABIH). The BCSP offers the Certified Safety Professional (CSP) credential, while the ABIH proffers the Certified Industrial Hygienist (CIH) credential. Also, the Council on Certification of Health, Environmental, and Safety Technologists, a joint effort between the BCSP and ABIH, awards the Occupational Health and Safety Technologist (OHST) credential.

Requirements for the OHST credential are less stringent than those for the CSP or CIH credentials. Once education and experience requirements have been met, certification may be obtained through an examination. Continuing education is required for recertification. Although voluntary, many employers encourage certification. Federal Government occupational health and safety specialists and technicians whose job performance is satisfactory advance through their career ladder to a specified full-performance level. For positions above this level, usually supervisory positions, advancement is competitive and based on agency needs and individual merit.

Advancement opportunities in State and local governments and the private sector are often similar to those in the Federal Government. With additional experience or education, promotion to a managerial position is possible. Research or related teaching positions at the college level require advanced education.

JOB OUTLOOK

Employment of occupational health and safety specialists and technicians is expected to grow about as fast as the average for all occupations through 2010, reflecting a balance of continuing public demand for a safe and healthy work environment against the desire for smaller government and fewer regulations. Additional job openings will arise from the need to replace those who transfer to other occupations, retire, or leave the labor force for other reasons. In private industry, employment growth will reflect industry growth and the continuing self- enforcement of government and company regulations and policies. Employment of occupational health and safety specialists and technicians is seldom affected by general economic fluctuations. Federal, State, and local governments, which employ almost half of all specialists and technicians, provide considerable job security.

EARNINGS

Median annual earnings of occupational health and safety specialists and technicians were $42,750 in 2000. The middle 50 percent earned between $32,060 and $54,880. The lowest 10 percent earned less than $23,780, while the highest 10 percent earned over $67,760. Median annual earnings of occupational health and safety specialists and technicians in 2000 were $41,330 in local government and $41,110 in State government. Most occupational health and safety specialists and technicians work for Federal, State, and local governments or in large private firms, most of which generally offer more generous benefits than do smaller firms.

RELATED OCCUPATIONS

Occupational health and safety specialists and technicians ensure that laws and regulations are obeyed. Others who enforce laws and regulations include agricultural inspectors, construction and building inspectors, correctional officers, financial examiners, fire inspectors, police and detectives, and transportation inspectors.

SOURCES OF ADDITIONAL INFORMATION

Information about jobs in Federal, State, and local government as well as in private industry is available from the States' employment service offices.

For information on a career as an industrial hygienist and a list of colleges and universities offering programs in industrial hygiene, contact: American Industrial Hygiene Association, 2700 Prosperity Ave., Suite 250, Fairfax, VA 22031. Internet: http://www.aiha.org

For a list of colleges and universities offering safety and related degrees, including correspondence courses, contact: American Society of Safety Engineers, 1800 E Oakton St., Des Plaines, IL 60018. Internet: http://www.asse.org

For information on the Certified Safety Professional credential, contact: Board of Certified Safety Professionals, 208 Burwash Ave., Savoy, IL 61874. Internet: http://www.bcsp.org

For information on the Certified Industrial Hygiene credential, contact: American Board of Industrial Hygiene, 6015 West St. Joseph, Suite 102, Lansing, MI 48917. Internet: http://www.abih.org

For information on the Occupational Health and Safety Technologist credential, contact: Council on Certification of Health, Environmental, and Safety Technologists, 208 Burwash Ave., Savoy, IL 61874. Internet: http://www.cchest.org

For additional career information, contact:

- U.S. Department of Health and Human Services, Center for Disease Control and Prevention, National Institute of Occupational Safety and Health, Hubert H. Humphrey Bldg., 200 Independence Ave. SW., Room 715H, Washington, DC 20201. Internet: http://www.cdc.gov/niosh/homepage.html

- U.S. Department of Labor, Occupational Safety and Health Administration, 200 Constitution Ave. NW., Washington, DC 20210. Internet: http://www.osha.gov

Information on obtaining positions as occupational health and safety specialists and technicians with the Federal Government is available from the Office of Personnel Management through a telephone-based system. Consult your telephone directory under U.S. Government for a local number or call (912) 757-3000; Federal Relay Service: (800) 877-8339. The first number is not tollfree, and charges may result. Information also is available from the Internet site: http://www.usajobs.opm.gov.

Chapter 25

OPTICIANS, DISPENSING

SIGNIFICANT POINTS

- Most dispensing opticians receive training on-the-job or through apprenticeships lasting 2 or more years; 22 States require a license.
- Projected employment growth reflects steadfast demand for corrective lenses and trends in fashion.
- The number of job openings will be relatively small because the occupation is small.

NATURE OF WORK

Dispensing opticians fit eyeglasses and contact lenses, following prescriptions written by ophthalmologists or optometrists. Dispensing opticians examine written prescriptions to determine lens specifications. They recommend eyeglass frames, lenses, and lens coatings after considering the prescription and the customer's occupation, habits, and facial features. Dispensing opticians measure clients' eyes, including the distance between the centers of the pupils and the distance between the eye surface and the lens. For customers without prescriptions, dispensing opticians may use a lensometer to record the present eyeglass prescription. They also may obtain a customer's previous record, or verify a prescription with the examining optometrist or ophthalmologist. Dispensing opticians prepare work orders that give ophthalmic laboratory technicians information needed to grind and insert lenses into a frame. The work order includes lens prescriptions and information on lens size, material, color, and style.

Some dispensing opticians grind and insert lenses themselves. After the glasses are made, dispensing opticians verify that the lenses have been ground to specifications. Then they may reshape or bend the frame, by hand or using pliers, so that the eyeglasses fit the customer properly and comfortably. Some also fix, adjust, and refit broken frames. They instruct clients about adapting to, wearing, or caring for eyeglasses.

Some dispensing opticians specialize in fitting contacts, artificial eyes, or cosmetic shells to cover blemished eyes. To fit contact lenses, dispensing opticians measure eye shape and size, select the type of contact lens material, and prepare work orders specifying the prescription and lens size. Fitting contact lenses requires considerable skill, care, and patience.

Dispensing opticians observe customers' eyes, corneas, lids, and contact lenses with special instruments and microscopes. During several visits, opticians show customers how to insert, remove, and care for their contacts, and ensure the fit is correct. Dispensing opticians keep records on customer prescriptions, work orders, and payments; track inventory and sales; and perform other administrative duties.

WORKING CONDITIONS

Dispensing opticians work indoors in attractive, well-lighted, and well-ventilated surroundings. They may work in medical offices or small stores where customers are served one at a time, or in large stores where several dispensing opticians serve a number of customers at once. Opticians spend a lot of time on their feet. If they prepare lenses, they need to take precautions against the hazards associated with glass cutting, chemicals, and machinery. Most dispensing opticians work a 40-hour week, although some work longer hours. Those in retail stores may work evenings and weekends. Some work part time.

EMPLOYMENT

Dispensing opticians held about 68,000 jobs in 2000. Almost half worked for ophthalmologists or optometrists who sell glasses directly to patients. Many also work in retail optical stores that offer one-stop shopping.

Customers may have their eyes examined, choose frames, and have glasses made on the spot. Some work in optical departments of drug and department stores.

TRAINING, OTHER QUALIFICATIONS AND ADVANCEMENT

Employers usually hire individuals with no background in opticianry or those who have worked as ophthalmic laboratory technicians and then provide the required training. Most dispensing opticians receive training on-the-job or through apprenticeships lasting 2 or more years.

Some employers, however, seek people with postsecondary training in opticianry. Knowledge of physics, basic anatomy, algebra, geometry, and mechanical drawing is particularly valuable because training usually includes instruction in optical mathematics, optical physics, and the use of precision measuring instruments and other machinery and tools. Dispensing opticians deal directly with the public, so they should be tactful, pleasant, and communicate well. Manual dexterity and the ability to do precision work are essential. Large employers usually offer structured apprenticeship programs, and small employers provide more informal on-the-job training.

In the 22 States that require dispensing opticians to be licensed, individuals without postsecondary training work from 2 to 4 years as apprentices. Apprenticeship or formal training is offered in most States as well. Apprentices receive technical training and learn office management and sales. Under the supervision of an experienced optician, optometrist, or ophthalmologist, apprentices work directly with patients, fitting eyeglasses and contact lenses.

In the 21 States requiring licensure, information about apprenticeships and licensing procedures is available from the State board of occupational licensing. Formal opticianry training is offered in community colleges and a few colleges and universities. In 2000, the Commission on Opticianry Accreditation accredited 25 programs that awarded 2-year associate degrees in opticianry. There also are shorter programs of 1 year or less.

Some States that offer a license to dispensing opticians allow graduates to take the licensure exam immediately upon graduation; others require a few months to a year of experience. Dispensing opticians may apply to the American Board of Opticianry (ABO) and the National Contact Lens Examiners (NCLE) for certification of their skills. Certification must be renewed every 3 years through continuing education. Those licensed in States where licensing renewal requirements include continuing education credits may use proof of their renewed State license to meet the recertification requirements of the ABO. Likewise, the NCLE will accept proof of license renewal from any State that has contact lens requirements.

Many experienced dispensing opticians open their own optical stores. Others become managers of optical stores or sales representatives for wholesalers or manufacturers of eyeglasses or lenses.

JOB OUTLOOK

Employment of dispensing opticians is expected to increase about as fast as the average for all occupations through 2010 as demand grows for corrective lenses. The number of middle-aged and elderly persons is projected to increase rapidly. Middle age is a time when many individuals use corrective lenses for the first time, and elderly persons generally require more vision care than others. Fashion, too, influences demand. Frames come in a growing variety of styles and colors-encouraging people to buy more than one pair. Demand also is expected to grow in response to the availability of new technologies that improve the quality and look of corrective lenses, such as anti-reflective coatings and bifocal lenses without the line visible in old-style bifocals. Improvements in bifocal, extended wear, and disposable contact lenses also will spur demand. The need to replace those who leave the occupation will result in additional job openings. Nevertheless, the total number of job openings will be relatively small because the occupation is small. This occupation is vulnerable to changes in the business cycle because eyewear purchases often can be deferred for a time. Employment of opticians can fall somewhat during economic downturns.

EARNINGS

Median annual earnings of dispensing opticians were $24,430 in 2000. The middle 50 percent earned between $19,200 and $31,770. The lowest 10 percent earned less than $15,900, and the highest 10 percent earned more than $39,660. Median annual earnings in the industries employing the largest numbers of dispensing opticians in 2000 were as follows:

- Offices and clinics of medical doctors $28,220
- Retail stores, not elsewhere classified $25,120
- Offices of other health practitioners $22,670
- Department stores $21,410

RELATED OCCUPATIONS

Other workers who deal with customers and perform delicate work include camera and photographic equipment repairers, dental laboratory technicians, jewelers and precious stone and metal workers, locksmiths and safe repairers, ophthalmic laboratory technicians, orthotists and prosthetists, and watch repairers.

SOURCES OF ADDITIONAL INFORMATION

For general information about a career as a dispensing optician and about continuing education, as well as a list of State licensing boards for opticianry, contact: Opticians Association of America, 7023 Little River Turnpike, Suite 207, Annandale, VA 22003. Internet: http://www.opticians.org

For general information about a career as a dispensing optician and a list of accredited training programs, contact: Commission on Opticianry Accreditation, 7023 Little River Turnpike, Suite 207, Annandale, VA 22003. Internet: http://www.coaccreditation.com

For general information on opticianry and a list of home-study programs, seminars, and review materials, contact: National Academy of Opticianry, 8401 Corporate Dr., Suite 605, Landover, MD 20785. Internet: http://www.nao.org

To learn about voluntary certification for opticians who fit spectacles, as well as State licensing boards of opticianry, contact: American Board of Opticianry, 6506 Loisdale Rd., Suite 209, Springfield, VA 22150. Internet: http://www.abo.org

For information on voluntary certification for dispensing opticians who fit contact lenses, contact: National Contact Lens Examiners, 6506 Loisdale Rd., Suite 209, Springfield, VA 22150. Internet: http://www.abo.org

Chapter 26

PHARMACY TECHNICIANS

SIGNIFICANT POINTS

- Job opportunities are expected to be good, especially for those with certification or previous work experience.
- Many technicians work evenings, weekends, and some holidays.
- Two-thirds of all jobs are in retail pharmacies.

NATURE OF THE WORK

Pharmacy technicians help licensed pharmacists provide medication and other healthcare products to patients. Technicians usually perform routine tasks to help prepare prescribed medication for patients, such as counting tablets and labeling bottles. Technicians refer any questions regarding prescriptions, drug information, or health matters to a pharmacist.

Pharmacy aides work closely with pharmacy technicians. They are often clerks or cashiers who primarily answer telephones, handle money, stock shelves, and perform other clerical duties.

Pharmacy technicians usually perform more complex tasks than do pharmacy aides, although, in some States, their duties and job titles overlap. Pharmacy technicians who work in retail pharmacies have varying responsibilities, depending on State rules and regulations. Technicians receive written prescriptions or requests for prescription refills from patients. They also may receive prescriptions sent electronically from the doctor's office. They must verify that the information on the prescription is complete and accurate.

To prepare the prescription, technicians must retrieve, count, pour, weigh, measure, and sometimes mix the medication. Then, they prepare the prescription labels, select the type of prescription container, and affix the prescription and auxiliary labels to the container. Once the prescription is filled, technicians price and file the prescription, which must be checked by a pharmacist before it is given to a patient.

Technicians may establish and maintain patient profiles, prepare insurance claim forms, and stock and take inventory of prescription and over-the-counter medications.

In hospitals, technicians have added responsibilities. They read patient charts and prepare and deliver the medicine to patients. The pharmacist must check the order before it is delivered to the patient. The technician then copies the information about the prescribed medication onto the patient's profile. Technicians also may assemble a 24-hour supply of medicine for every patient. They package and label each dose separately. The package is then placed in the medicine cabinet of each patient until the supervising pharmacist checks it for accuracy. It is then given to the patient.

WORKING CONDITIONS

Pharmacy technicians work in clean, organized, well-lighted, and well-ventilated areas. Most of their workday is spent on their feet. They may be required to lift heavy boxes or to use stepladders to retrieve supplies from high shelves. Technicians work the same hours as pharmacists. This may include evenings, nights, weekends, and holidays. Because some hospital and retail pharmacies are open 24 hours a day, technicians may work varying shifts. As their seniority increases, technicians often have increased control over the hours they work. There are many opportunities for part-time work in both retail and hospital settings.

EMPLOYMENT

Pharmacy technicians held about 190,000 jobs in 2000. Two-thirds of all jobs were in retail pharmacies, either independently owned or part of a drug store chain, grocery store, department store, or mass retailer. More than

2 out of 10 jobs were in hospitals and a small number were in mail-order and Internet pharmacies, clinics, pharmaceutical wholesalers, and the Federal Government.

TRAINING, OTHER QUALIFICATIONS AND ADVANCEMENT

Although most pharmacy technicians receive informal on-the-job training, employers favor those who have completed formal training and certification. However, there are currently few State and no Federal requirements for formal training or certification of pharmacy technicians. Employers who can neither afford, nor have the time to give, on-the-job training often seek formally educated pharmacy technicians.

Formal education programs and certification emphasize the technicians' interest in and dedication to the work to potential employers. In addition to the military, some hospitals, proprietary schools, vocational or technical colleges, and community colleges offer formal education programs. Formal pharmacy-technician education programs require classroom and laboratory work in a variety of areas, including medical and pharmaceutical terminology, pharmaceutical calculations, pharmacy recordkeeping, pharmaceutical techniques, and pharmacy law and ethics.

Technicians also are required to learn medication names, actions, uses, and doses. Many training programs include internships, in which students gain hands-on experience in actual pharmacies. Students receive a diploma, certificate, or an associate degree, depending on the program. Prospective pharmacy technicians with experience working as an aide in a community pharmacy or volunteering in a hospital may have an advantage. Employers also prefer applicants with strong customer service and communication skills and with experience managing inventories, counting, measuring, and using computers.

Technicians entering the field need strong mathematics, spelling, and reading skills. A background in chemistry, English, and health education also may be beneficial. Some technicians are hired without formal training, but under the condition that they obtain certification within a specified period to retain employment.

The Pharmacy Technician Certification Board administers the National Pharmacy Technician Certification Examination. This exam is voluntary and displays the competency of the individual to act as a pharmacy technician.

Eligible candidates must have a high school diploma or GED, and those who pass the exam earn the title of Certified Pharmacy Technician (CPhT). The exam is offered several times per year at various locations nationally. Employers, often pharmacists, know that individuals who pass the exam have a standardized body of knowledge and skills. Certified technicians must be recertified every 2 years. Technicians must complete 20 contact hours of pharmacy-related topics within the 2-year certification period to become eligible for recertification. Contact hours are awarded for on-the-job training, attending lectures, and college coursework. At least 1 contact hour must be in pharmacy law. Contact hours can be earned from several different sources, including pharmacy associations, pharmacy colleges, and pharmacy technician training programs. Up to 10 contact hours can be earned when the technician is employed under the direct supervision and instruction of a pharmacist.

Successful pharmacy technicians are alert, observant, organized, dedicated, and responsible. They should be willing and able to take directions. They must enjoy precise work-details are sometimes a matter of life and death. Although a pharmacist must check and approve all their work, they should be able to work on their own without constant instruction from the pharmacist. Candidates interested in becoming pharmacy technicians cannot have prior records of drug or substance abuse. Strong interpersonal and communication skills are needed because there is a lot of interaction with patients, coworkers, and healthcare professionals. Teamwork is very important because technicians are often required to work with pharmacists, aides, and other technicians.

JOB OUTLOOK

Good job opportunities are expected for full-time and part-time work, especially for technicians with formal training or previous experience. Job openings for pharmacy technicians will result from the expansion of retail pharmacies and other employment settings, and from the need to replace workers who transfer to other occupations or leave the labor force. Employment of pharmacy technicians is expected to grow much faster than the average for all occupations through 2010 due to the increased pharmaceutical needs of a larger and older population, and to the greater use of medication. The increased number of middle-aged and elderly people-who, on average, use more prescription drugs than do younger people-will spur demand for technicians in all practice settings. With advances in science, more medications are becoming available to treat more conditions. Cost-conscious insurers, pharmacies, and health systems will continue to emphasize the role of technicians. As a result, pharmacy technicians will assume responsibility for more routine tasks previously performed by pharmacists. Pharmacy technicians also will need to learn and master new pharmacy technology as it surfaces. For example, robotic machines are used to dispense medicine into containers; technicians must oversee the machines, stock the bins, and label the containers. Thus, while automation is increasingly incorporated into the job, it will not necessarily reduce the need for technicians. Almost all States have legislated the maximum number of technicians who can safely work under a pharmacist at a time. In some States, increased demand for technicians has encouraged an expanded ratio of technicians to pharmacists. Changes in these laws could directly affect employment.

EARNINGS

Median hourly earnings of pharmacy technicians in 2000 were $9.93. The middle 50 percent earned between $8.12 and $12.26; the lowest 10 percent earned less than $7.00, and the highest 10 percent earned more than $14.56. Median hourly earnings in the industries employing the largest numbers of pharmacy technicians in 2000 were as follows:

- Hospitals $11.44
- Grocery stores $10.57
- Drugs, proprietaries, and sundries $10.09
- Drug stores and proprietary stores $9.00
- Department stores $8.75

Certified technicians may earn more. Shift differentials for working evenings or weekends also can increase earnings. Some technicians belong to unions representing hospital or grocery store workers.

RELATED OCCUPATIONS

This occupation is most closely related to pharmacists and pharmacy aides. Workers in other medical support occupations include dental assistants, licensed practical and licensed vocational nurses, medical transcriptionists, medical records and health information technicians, occupational therapist assistants and aides, physical therapist assistants and aides, secretaries and administrative assistants, and surgical technologists.

SOURCES OF ADDITIONAL INFORMATION

For information on certification and a National Pharmacy Technician Certification Examination Candidate Handbook, contact: Pharmacy Technician Certification Board, 2215 Constitution Ave. NW., Washington DC 20037. Internet: http://www.ptcb.org

Chapter 27

RADIOLOGIC TECHNOLOGISTS AND TECHNICIANS

SIGNIFICANT POINTS

- Faster-than-average growth will arise from an increase in the number of middle-aged and older persons who are the primary users of diagnostic procedures
- Although hospitals will remain the primary employer of radiologic technologists and technicians, a greater number of new jobs will be found in offices and clinics of physicians, including diagnostic imaging centers.
- Radiologic technologists and technicians with cross training in nuclear medicine technology or other modalities will have the best prospects.

NATURE OF THE WORK

Radiologic technologists and technicians take x rays and administer nonradioactive materials into patients' blood streams for diagnostic purposes. Some specialize in diagnostic imaging technologies such as computed tomography (CT) and magnetic resonance imaging (MRI). In addition to radiologic technologists and technicians, others who assist in diagnostic imaging procedures include cardiovascular technologists and technicians, diagnostic medical sonographers, and nuclear medicine technologists.

Radiologic technologists and technicians, also referred to as radiographers, produce x-ray films (radiographs) of parts of the human body for use in diagnosing medical problems. They prepare patients for radiologic examinations by explaining the procedure, removing articles such as jewelry, through which x rays cannot pass, and positioning patients so that the parts of the body can be appropriately radiographed. To prevent unnecessary radiation exposure, they surround the exposed area with radiation protection devices, such as lead shields, or limit the size of the x-ray beam. Radiographers position radiographic equipment at the correct angle and height over the appropriate area of a patient's body. Using instruments similar to a measuring tape, they may measure the thickness of the section to be radiographed and set controls on the x-ray machine to produce radiographs of the appropriate density, detail, and contrast. They place the x-ray film under the part of the patient's body to be examined and make the exposure. They then remove the film and develop it. Experienced radiographers may perform more complex imaging procedures. For fluoroscopies, radiographers prepare a solution of contrast medium for the patient to drink, allowing the radiologist, a physician who interprets radiographs, to see soft tissues in the body.

Some radiographers, called CT technologists, operate computerized tomography scanners to produce cross sectional images of patients. Others operate machines using strong magnets and radio waves rather than radiation to create an image and are called magnetic resonance imaging (MRI) technologists.

Radiologic technologists and technicians must follow physicians' orders precisely and conform to regulations concerning use of radiation to protect themselves, their patients, and coworkers from unnecessary exposure. In addition to preparing patients and operating equipment, radiologic technologists and technicians keep patient records and adjust and maintain equipment. They also may prepare work schedules, evaluate equipment purchases, or manage a radiology department.

WORKING CONDITIONS

Most full-time radiologic technologists and technicians work about 40 hours a week; they may have evening, weekend, or on-call hours. Opportunities for part-time and shift work are also available. Because technologists and technicians are on their feet for long periods and may lift or turn disabled patients, physical stamina is important. Technologists and technicians work at diagnostic machines but may also do some procedures at patients' bedsides. Some travel to patients in large vans equipped with sophisticated diagnostic equipment. Although potential radiation hazards exist in this occupation, they are minimized by the use of lead aprons, gloves, and other shielding devices, as well as by instruments monitoring radiation exposure. Technologists and technicians wear badges measuring radiation levels in the radiation area, and detailed records are kept on their cumulative lifetime dose.

EMPLOYMENT

Radiologic technologists and technicians held about 167,000 jobs in 2000. About 1 in 5 worked part time. More than half of all jobs are in hospitals. Most of the rest are in physicians' offices and clinics, including diagnostic imaging centers.

TRAINING, OTHER QUALIFICATIONS AND ADVANCEMENT

Preparation for this profession is offered in hospitals, colleges and universities, vocational-technical institutes, and the U.S. Armed Forces. Hospitals, which employ most radiologic technologists and technicians, prefer to hire those with formal training.

Formal training programs in radiography range in length from 1 to 4 years and lead to a certificate, associate's degree, or bachelor's degree. Two-year associate's degree programs are most prevalent. Some 1-year certificate programs are available for experienced radiographers or individuals from other health occupations, such as medical technologists and registered nurses, who want to change fields or specialize in computerized tomography or magnetic resonance imaging. A bachelor's or master's degree in one of the radiologic technologies is desirable for supervisory, administrative, or teaching positions.

The Joint Review Committee on Education in Radiologic Technology accredits most formal training programs for this field. They accredited 584 radiography programs in 2000. Radiography programs require, at a minimum, a high school diploma or the equivalent. High school courses in mathematics, physics, chemistry, and biology are helpful. The programs provide both classroom and clinical instruction in anatomy and physiology, patient care procedures, radiation physics, radiation protection, principles of imaging, medical terminology, positioning of patients, medical ethics, radiobiology, and pathology.

In 1981, Congress passed the Consumer-Patient Radiation Health and Safety Act, which aims to protect the public from the hazards of unnecessary exposure to medical and dental radiation by ensuring operators of radiologic equipment are properly trained. Under the act, the Federal Government sets voluntary standards that the States, in turn, may use for accrediting training programs and certifying individuals who engage in medical or dental radiography.

In 1999, 35 States and Puerto Rico licensed radiologic technologists and technicians. Voluntary registration is offered by the American Registry of Radiologic Technologists (ARRT) in radiography. To be eligible for registration, technologists generally must graduate from an accredited program and pass an examination. Many employers prefer to hire registered radiographers. To be recertified, radiographers must complete 24 hours of continuing education every other year.

Radiologic technologists and technicians should be sensitive to patients' physical and psychological needs. They must pay attention to detail, follow instructions, and work as part of a team. In addition, operating complicated equipment requires mechanical ability and manual dexterity. With experience and additional training, staff technologists may become specialists, performing CT scanning, angiography, and magnetic resonance imaging.

Experienced technologists may also be promoted to supervisor, chief radiologic technologist, and-ultimately-department administrator or director. Depending on the institution, courses or a master's degree in business or health administration may be necessary for the director's position. Some technologists progress by becoming instructors or directors in radiologic technology programs; others take jobs as sales representatives or instructors with equipment manufacturers.

JOB OUTLOOK

Employment of radiologic technologists and technicians is expected to grow faster than the average for all occupations through 2010, as the population grows and ages, increasing the demand for diagnostic imaging. Opportunities are expected to be favorable. Some employers report shortages of radiologic technologists and technicians. Imbalances between the supply of qualified workers and demand should spur efforts to attract and retain qualified radiologic technologists and technicians. For example, employers may provide more flexible training programs, or improve compensation and working conditions. Although physicians are enthusiastic about the clinical benefits of new technologies, the extent to which they are adopted depends largely on cost and reimbursement considerations. For example, digital imaging technology can improve quality and efficiency, but remains expensive. Some promising new technologies may not come into widespread use because they are too expensive and third-party payers may not be willing to pay for their use.

Radiologic technologists who are educated and credentialed in more than one type of diagnostic imaging technology, such as radiography and sonography or nuclear medicine, will have better employment opportunities as employers look for new ways to control costs. In hospitals, multi-skilled employees will be the most sought after, as hospitals respond to cost pressures by continuing to merge departments. Hospitals will remain the principal employer of radiologic technologists and technicians. However, a greater number of new jobs will be found in offices and clinics of physicians, including diagnostic imaging centers. Health facilities such as these are expected to grow very rapidly through 2010 due to the strong shift toward outpatient care, encouraged by third-party payers and made possible by technological advances that permit more procedures to be performed outside the hospital. Some job openings will also arise from the need to replace technologists and technicians who leave the occupation.

EARNINGS

Median annual earnings of radiologic technologists and technicians were $36,000 in 2000. The middle 50 percent earned between $30,220 and $43,380. The lowest 10 percent earned less than $25,310, and the highest 10 percent earned more than $52,050. Median annual earnings in the industries employing the largest numbers of radiologic technologists and technicians in 2000 were:

- Medical and dental laboratories $39,400
- Hospitals $36,280
- Offices and clinics of medical doctors $34,870

RELATED OCCUPATIONS

Radiologic technologists and technicians operate sophisticated equipment to help physicians, dentists, and other health practitioners diagnose and treat patients. Workers in related occupations include cardiovascular technologists and technicians, clinical laboratory technologists and technicians, diagnostic medical sonographers, nuclear medicine technologists, radiation therapists, and respiratory therapists.

SOURCES OF ADDITIONAL INFORMATION

For career information, send a stamped, self-addressed business size envelope with your request to: American Society of Radiologic Technologists, 15000 Central Ave. SE., Albuquerque, NM 87123-3917. Internet: http://www.asrt.org/asrt.htm

For the current list of accredited education programs in radiography, write to: Joint Review Committee on Education in Radiologic Technology, 20 N. Wacker Dr., Suite 600, Chicago, IL 60606-2901. Internet: http://www.jrcert.org

For information on certification, contact: American Registry of Radiologic Technologists, 1255 Northland Dr., St. Paul, MN 55120-1155. Internet: http://www.arrt.org

Chapter 28

SURGICAL TECHNOLOGISTS

SIGNIFICANT POINTS

- Most educational programs for surgical technologists last approximately 1 year and result in a certificate.
- Employment of surgical technologists is expected to grow faster than average as the number of surgical procedures grows.

NATURE OF THE WORK

Surgical technologists, also called scrubs and surgical or operating room technicians, assist in surgical operations under the supervision of surgeons, registered nurses, or other surgical personnel. Surgical technologists are members of operating room teams, which most commonly include surgeons, anesthesiologists, and circulating nurses. Before an operation, surgical technologists help prepare the operating room by setting up surgical instruments and equipment, sterile drapes, and sterile solutions. They assemble both sterile and nonsterile equipment, as well as adjust and check it to ensure it is working properly.

Technologists also get patients ready for surgery by washing, shaving, and disinfecting incision sites. They transport patients to the operating room, help position them on the operating table, and cover them with sterile surgical "drapes." Technologists also observe patients' vital signs, check charts, and assist the surgical team with putting on sterile gowns and gloves. During surgery, technologists pass instruments and other sterile supplies to surgeons and surgeon assistants. They may hold retractors, cut sutures, and help count sponges, needles, supplies, and instruments.

Surgical technologists help prepare, care for, and dispose of specimens taken for laboratory analysis and help apply dressings. Some operate sterilizers, lights, or suction machines, and help operate diagnostic equipment. After an operation, surgical technologists may help transfer patients to the recovery room and clean and restock the operating room.

Working Conditions

Surgical technologists work in clean, well-lighted, cool environments. They must stand for long periods and remain alert during operations. At times they may be exposed to communicable diseases and unpleasant sights, odors, and materials. Most surgical technologists work a regular 40-hour week, although they may be on call or work nights, weekends and holidays on a rotating basis.

Employment

Surgical technologists held about 71,000 jobs in 2000. Almost three-quarters are employed by hospitals, mainly in operating and delivery rooms. Others are employed in clinics and surgical centers, and in the offices of physicians and dentists who perform outpatient surgery. A few, known as private scrubs, are employed directly by surgeons who have special surgical teams, like those for liver transplants.

Training, Other Qualifications and Advancement

Surgical technologists receive their training in formal programs offered by community and junior colleges, vocational schools, universities, hospitals, and the military. In 2001, the Commission on Accreditation of Allied Health Education Programs (CAAHEP) recognized 350 accredited programs. High school graduation normally is required for admission. Programs last 9 to 24 months and lead to a certificate, diploma, or associate degree. Programs provide classroom education and supervised clinical experience. Students take courses in anatomy, physiology, microbiology, pharmacology, professional ethics, and medical terminology. Other studies cover the care and safety of patients during surgery, aseptic techniques, and surgical procedures. Students also learn to sterilize instruments; prevent and control infection; and handle special drugs, solutions, supplies, and equipment.

Technologists may obtain voluntary professional certification from the Liaison Council on Certification for the Surgical Technologist by graduating from a CAAHEP-accredited program and passing a national certification examination. They may then use the designation Certified Surgical Technologist, or CST. Continuing education or reexamination is required to maintain certification, which must be renewed every 6 years.

Certification may also be obtained from the National Center for Competency Testing. To qualify to take the exam, candidates follow one of three paths: complete an accredited training program, undergo a 2-year hospital on-the-job training program, or acquire seven years experience working in the field. After passing the exam, individuals may use the designation National Certified Technician O.R. This certification may be renewed every 5 years through either continuing education or reexamination.

Most employers prefer to hire certified technologists. Surgical technologists need manual dexterity to handle instruments quickly. They also must be conscientious, orderly, and emotionally stable to handle the demands of the operating room environment.

Technologists must respond quickly and know procedures well to have instruments ready for surgeons without having to be told. They are expected to keep abreast of new developments in the field. Recommended high school courses include health, biology, chemistry, and mathematics. Technologists advance by specializing in a particular area of surgery, such as neurosurgery or open heart surgery. They also may work as circulating technologists. A circulating technologist is the "unsterile" member of the surgical team who prepares patients; helps with anesthesia; obtains and opens packages for the "sterile" persons to remove the sterile contents during the procedure; interviews the patient before surgery; keeps a written account of the surgical procedure; and answers the surgeon's questions about the patient during the surgery.

With additional training, some technologists advance to first assistants, who help with retracting, sponging, suturing, cauterizing bleeders, and closing and treating wounds. Some surgical technologists manage central supply departments in hospitals, or take positions with insurance companies, sterile supply services, and operating equipment firms.

JOB OUTLOOK

Employment of surgical technologists is expected to grow faster than the average for all occupations through the year 2010 as the volume of surgery increases. The number of surgical procedures is expected to rise as the population grows and ages. As the "baby boom" generation enters retirement age, the over 50 population will account for a larger portion of the general population. Older people require more surgical procedures. Technological advances, such as fiber optics and laser technology, will also permit new surgical procedures to be performed. Hospitals will continue to be the primary employer of surgical technologists, although much faster employment growth is expected in offices and clinics of physicians, including ambulatory surgical centers.

EARNINGS

Median annual earnings of surgical technologists were $29,020 in 2000. The middle 50 percent earned between $24,490 and $34,160. The lowest 10 percent earned less than $20,490, and the highest 10 percent earned more than $40,310. Median annual earnings of surgical technologists in 2000 were $31,190 in offices and clinics of medical doctors and $28,340 in hospitals.

RELATED OCCUPATIONS

Other health occupations requiring approximately 1 year of training after high school include dental assistants, licensed practical and licensed vocational nurses, medical and clinical laboratory technicians, medical assistants, and respiratory therapy technicians.

SOURCES OF ADDITIONAL INFORMATION

For additional information on a career as a surgical technologist and a list of CAAHEP-accredited programs, contact: Association of Surgical Technologists, 7108-C South Alton Way, Englewood, CO 80112. Internet: http://www.ast.org

For information on becoming a Certified Surgical Technologist, contact: Liaison Council on Certification for the Surgical Technologist, 7790 East Arapahoe Rd., Suite 240, Englewood, CO 80112-1274. Internet: http://www.lcc-st.org/index_ie.htm

For information on becoming a National Certified Technician O.R., contact: National Center for Competency Testing, 7007 College Blvd., Suite 250, Overland Park, KS 6621. Internet: http://www.ncctinc.com

INDEX

A

abdominal sonographers, 122
abstract reasoning, 20
academic medical centers, 48
accidents, 72, 127, 154
Accrediting Bureau of Health Education Schools (ABHES), 110
adaptive equipment, 20
adult daycare programs, 21, 41, 67, 68
advanced practice nurses, 71, 73
aging, 16, 28, 56, 75, 87, 89, 101, 131
agribusiness, 96
AIDS, 94, 129
air traffic controllers, 132
alcoholism, 20
allergic reactions, 36
Alliance of Cardiovascular Professionals, 106
allopathic physicians, 51, 57
alternative communication methods, 86
Alzheimer's disease, 72
ambulatory clinics, 75
ambulatory surgery centers, 104
American Academy of Physician Assistants, 46, 49
American Association for Respiratory Care, 84
American Association of Bioanalysts, 110, 113
American Association of Blood Banks, 113
American Association of Colleges of Nursing, 77
American Board of Industrial Hygiene (ABIH), 156, 158
American Board of Medical Specialists (ABMS), 56
American Board of Opticianry (ABO), 164, 166
American Chiropractic Association, 5, 6
American Dental Association Joint Commission on National Dental Examinations, 117
American Dental Association, 8, 9, 11, 118, 119
American Dental Hygienists' Association, 118
American Dietetic Association (ADA), 15, 17
American Health Information Management Association, 145
American Industrial Hygiene Association, 158

American Medical Association, 53, 57, 58, 143
American Medical Technologists, 110, 113
American Nurses Association, 77
American Optometric Association, 27, 29
American Osteopathic Association (AOA), 56, 58
American Physical Therapy Association, 41, 43
American Podiatric Medical Association, 63
American Registry of Diagnostic Medical Sonographers (ARDMS), 124
American Registry of Diagnostic Medical Sonographers, 104, 106, 124, 126
American Registry of Radiologic Technologists (ARRT), 149, 151, 176, 178
American Society for Clinical Laboratory Science, 113
American Society for Clinical Pathology, 110, 112, 113
American Society of Echocardiography, 106
American Society of Radiologic Technologists, 151, 178
American Society of Safety Engineers, 158
American Speech-Language-Hearing Association, 89, 90, 91
American Therapeutic Recreation Association, 69
American Veterinary Medical Association, 95, 99, 100
anatomy, 4, 9, 41, 47, 55, 61, 67, 74, 82, 88, 97, 117, 124, 137, 141, 143, 145, 163, 176, 181
anesthesia, 53, 80, 102, 181
anesthesiologists, 179
anesthesiology, 53, 61, 81, 97

anesthetics, 7, 73, 115
angiography, 176
animal health problems, 93
antibiotics, 7, 94
anxiety, 65
apprenticeships, 161, 163
arthritis, 39, 60
assisted living, 65, 66, 68
associate degree in nursing, (A.D.N.), 74
asthma, 32, 80
audiologic rehabilitation, 87
audiologists, 23, 29, 40, 43, 49, 58, 85, 87-91
audiology, 85, 87, 88, 91
automated devices, 86
automation, 108, 171

B

bachelor of science degree in nursing (B.S.N.), 74, 77
balloon angioplasty, 102
basic bedside care, 135
behavior patterns, 86
biochemistry, 4, 9, 15, 27, 47, 55, 96, 97
biomechanics, 41
blood banks, 109
blood gas analyzer, 80
blood pressure testing, 72
Board of Certified Safety Professionals (BCSP), 156, 158
brain injury, 86
breathing disorders, 79

C

cancer, 32, 72, 94, 142, 150
cardiac catheterization, 101, 104
cardiac rehabilitation centers, 104
cardiac sonographers, 102, 104
cardiographic technicians, 103
cardiology technologists, 101

cardiology, 52, 53, 97, 101, 104, 149, 150
cardiopulmonary care skills, 79, 83
cardiopulmonary diseases, 83
cardiopulmonary physical therapy, 40
cardiopulmonary procedures, 81
cardiovascular technologists, 101, 104, 105, 122, 126, 173, 178
catheterization labs, 103
cerebral palsy, 20, 39, 86
Certificate of Clinical Competence in Audiology (CCC-A), 89
Certificate of Clinical Competence in Speech-Language Pathology (CCC-SLP), 89
Certified Industrial Hygienist (CIH), 156
Certified Pharmacy Technician (CPhT), 170
Certified Respiratory Therapist (CRT), 82
Certified Safety Professional (CSP), 156, 158
Certified Surgical Technologist (CST), 181, 183
certified therapeutic recreation specialists (CTRS), 68
chemistry, 4, 9, 15, 22, 27, 34, 41, 47, 55, 61, 74, 82, 95, 108, 110, 117, 143, 156, 169, 176, 181
chemotherapy, 32, 76
chest physiotherapy, 80
childbirth, 72, 127, 130
childcare, 72, 77
chiropractic institutions, 3
chiropractic treatment, 5
chiropractors, 1-5, 11, 23, 29, 58, 63, 100
chronic bronchitis, 83
Clinical Competency Test (CCT), 97
clinical dental hygiene, 117
clinical dietitians, 14
Clinical Laboratory Improvement Act (CLIA), 110
clinical laboratory personnel, 110, 113
clinical laboratory technicians, 107, 110, 112, 182
clinical laboratory technologists, 107-112, 126, 151, 178
clinical laboratory workers, 111
clinical practice, 46, 49, 73, 79, 82, 93, 117, 137
Commission on Accreditation for Dietetics Education (CADE), 15
Commission on Accreditation of Allied Health Education Programs (CAAHEP), 110, 143, 145, 180-182
Commission on Opticianry Accreditation, 164, 165
Committee on Accreditation for Respiratory Care (CoARC), 82, 84
communicable diseases, 180
communication skills, 9, 34, 85, 86, 137, 169, 170
community centers, 73
community health education, 72
community integration programs, 67
community mental health centers, 21, 67
community settings, 21, 72
computed tomography (CT), 173, 174, 176
computerized tomography, 174, 175
Consumer-Patient Radiation Health and Safety Act, 176
contact lenses, 25, 26, 28, 161-164, 166
correctional facilities, 14, 15, 67
corrective surgery, 7
Council on Chiropractic Education, 3, 6
cystic fibrosis, 80
cytotechnologists, 108

D

daily life, 20
Dental Admissions Test (DAT), 9
dental assistants, 8, 10, 118, 172, 182
dental care, 7, 10, 98, 115, 117
dental hygienists, 8, 10, 115-118
dental schools, 9, 11
dental technology, 10
dentists, 5, 7-10, 29, 40, 46, 58, 63, 100, 117, 178, 180
Department of Labor, 155, 159
depression, 20, 65
dermatology, 60, 97
diabetes, 26, 28, 32, 59, 60
diabetics, 60
diagnosis-related groups (DRGs), 142
diagnostic imaging centers, 148, 175, 177
diagnostic imaging, 2, 3, 121, 123, 125, 147, 173, 176, 177
diagnostic medical sonographers, 122, 125
diagnostic medical sonography, 124
diagnostic tests, 51, 53, 111, 115
diet, 1, 7, 13-15, 51, 116
dietary habits, 16
dietetics, 13, 15-17
dietitians, 13-17
digital imaging technology, 177
direct patient care, 34, 49, 71
disabilities, 20, 22, 39, 42, 43, 65-69, 76, 89, 138
disabled students, 23, 66
disease management, 35
disease prevention, 13, 16, 47, 72
dispensing opticians, 26, 161, 162, 163, 164, 165, 166
Doctor of Chiropractic (DC), 3, 4, 11, 58, 77, 100, 133, 158, 159, 172
Doctor of Dental Medicine (DMD), 9
Doctor of Dental Surgery (DDS), 9
Doctor of Medicine (M.D.), 51, 53-57

Doctor of Medicine, 51, 55
Doctor of Optometry, 25, 27
Doctor of Osteopathic Medicine (D.O.), 51, 53-56
Doctor of Pharmacy (Pharm.D), 33, 34
Doctor of Pharmacy, 33
doctor of podiatric medicine, 61
Doctor of Veterinary Medicine (D.V.M. or V.M.D.), 95, 97
doctors of optometry (ODs), 25
doctors of podiatric medicine (DPMs), 59, 61, 62
drug abuse, 20, 68, 94
drug dispensing, 35
drug therap(ies), 31-33, 35, 94

E

earnings, vii, 1, 5, 10, 17, 23, 29, 36, 43, 48, 49, 51, 57, 59, 63, 69, 76, 83, 90, 99, 105, 111, 112, 118, 132, 138, 144, 150, 165, 171, 177, 182
eating disorders, 20
eating habits, 13
echocardiographers, 102, 105, 122
echocardiography, 101, 104, 106, 122
Educational Commission for Foreign Veterinary Graduates (ECFVG), 97
EKG technicians, 101, 104, 105
elderly, 10, 14, 19, 20, 26, 35, 39, 42, 62, 76, 80, 83, 137, 147, 164, 170
electrical stimulation, 40
electrocardiograms (EKGs), 81, 101, 104, 129
emergency care, 72, 80, 128
emergency medical centers, 72, 76, 137
emergency medical service(s) (EMS), 128-130, 132, 133
emergency medical technicians (EMTs), 47, 77, 127-133, 138

emergency medicine, 46-48, 53, 61
emergency visits, 54, 80
emotional problems, 86
emphysema, 80, 83
employment growth, 7, 10, 16, 35, 68, 90, 98, 144, 157, 161, 182
EMT-Basic (EMT-1), 128, 130, 131
EMT-Cardiac, 131
EMT-Intermediate (EMT-2/EMT-3), 128, 130-132
EMT-Paramedic (EMT-4), 128-131, 132
endodontists, 8
endotracheal intubations, 129
epidemiologists, 98
epidemiology, 99
exercise(s), 1, 2, 19, 40, 42, 66
eye diseases, 25, 26
eye surgery, 25, 26

F

family medicine, 46, 53
family practice, 28, 52, 55
family practitioners, 53, 56
federal agencies, 97
Federal Government, 15, 33, 54, 95, 99, 109, 118, 153, 155-157, 159, 169, 176
financial aid, 11, 29, 37, 58, 63, 100
financial assistance, 56
firefighting, 132
first aid, 137
first responders, 128
fitness workers, 65, 69
fluoroscopies, 174
food animals, 94, 99
food safety, 94, 99
food service managers, 14, 16, 17
food service systems, 13, 15
footcare, 59, 60, 62

G

general internal medicine, 53
general internists, 56
general pediatricians, 56
genetic disorders, 87
geriatrics, 4, 40, 46, 47, 60
group medical practices, 51, 57, 62
group practices, 54, 59, 60, 63, 94, 95, 143, 144
group practitioners, 2
gynecology, 47, 52, 53, 55, 57, 124

H

head injuries, 39
Health and Human Services, 54, 95, 155, 158
health care personnel, 141
health counseling, 72
health educators, 16, 17, 71
health information coders, 142
health information technicians, 141, 142, 143, 144, 145
health insurance, 5, 11, 62, 63
health maintenance organizations (HMOs), 14, 27
health practitioners, 2, 21, 23, 26, 29, 31, 43, 46, 60, 73, 90, 105, 118, 126, 151, 165, 178
health services industry, 48
healthcare facilities, 14, 73, 85, 123
healthcare networks, 54
hearing aids, 87
hearing disorders, 8-91
hearing loss, 86, 87, 89, 129
hearing protection programs, 87
hearing, 85-90, 129
heart attack(s), 22, 42, 80, 83, 127
heart disease, 39, 60, 83, 116
Hepatitis-B, 129
high blood pressure, 13, 26, 32
histology technicians, 108
histology, 117

holistic patient care, 51
Holter monitor(s), 101, 103
home health agencies, 14, 21, 41, 75, 79, 88, 141, 143, 144
home health aides, 72
home healthcare, 16, 21, 22, 32, 33, 46, 47, 68, 73, 76, 136, 138
hospital trauma centers, 128
human health problems, 94, 99
human immune system, 108

I

immunizations, 72
immunohematology technologists, 108
immunology, 56
independent laboratories, 109
industrial hygienists, 153
industrial nurses, 72
infants, 79, 83, 122, 136
infectious diseases, 7, 73, 81, 116, 136
injuries, 5, 26, 29, 39, 42, 45, 53, 58, 59, 63, 72, 73, 100, 128, 129, 136, 154
inoculations, 72
integrated healthcare networks, 76
integrated healthcare systems, 51, 57
intensive care, 56, 72, 82, 98
internal disorders, 2, 3
internal medicine, 46, 48, 53, 55, 57, 61, 97
interpersonal skills, 22, 42, 62, 124

J

job opportunities, 7, 10, 45, 121, 170
job prospects, 1, 56, 99, 105, 144
job training services, 21
jobs, 3, 7, 8, 10, 15, 21, 26, 33, 41, 46, 48, 54, 56, 57, 60, 67-69, 71, 73, 75, 81, 82, 88, 95, 98, 101, 104, 105, 109, 110, 116, 123, 129, 132, 135-137, 143, 148, 155, 158, 163, 167, 168, 173, 175-177, 180
Joint Review Committee on Education for Diagnostic Medical Sonography, 124
Joint Review Committee on Education in Cardiovascular Technology, 104, 106
Joint Review Committee on Education in Radiologic Technology, 175, 178

L

laboratory tests, 2, 45, 60, 107, 111, 135, 141
language skills, 86
language, 23, 29, 40, 43, 49, 58, 85-91, 97
laser surgery, 28
laser vision correction, 25
lensometer, 161
Liaison Council on Certification for the Surgical Technologist, 181, 183
licensed practical nurses (LPNs), 71, 72, 135-138
licensed vocational nurses (LVNs), 135, 172, 182
life insurance, 11
life support systems, 80
local anesthetics, 116
long-term care, 67, 76, 137
low back pain, 39
lung capacity, 80
lung diseases, 80

M

magnetic resonance imaging (MRI), 121, 173, 174, 175, 176
managed care organizations, 32, 62
manual defibrillators, 128
maternity, 72, 75

median annual earnings, 83, 90, 125, 157
Medicaid, 88
medical assistants, 45, 118, 182
Medical College Admission Test (MCAT), 55, 61, 96
medical education, 47, 55, 56
medical ethics, 47, 55, 124, 176
medical histories, 39, 45, 51, 55
medical records and health information technicians, 141, 143, 144, 172
medical school(s), 47, 55, 56, 58, 81, 95
medical secretaries, 145
medical technologists, 107, 149, 151, 175
medical technology, 42, 107-110
medical terminology, 141, 143, 145, 176, 181
medical transcriptionists, 145, 172
medical-surgical nursing, 137
Medicare, 144, 88
medication distribution systems, 35
medication interactions, 36
memory, 9, 20, 86
mental disorders, 32
mental retardation, 86
microbiology, 4, 9, 15, 47, 55, 74, 82, 96, 108, 110, 117, 181
motor functioning, 65
muscular dystrophy, 20
musculoskeletal system, 51
music therapy, 67

N

National Academy of Opticianry, 165
National Accrediting Agency for Clinical Laboratory Sciences (NAACLS), 110, 113
National Association for Practical Nurse Education and Service, 139
National Association of Boards of Pharmacy, 37
National Association of Emergency Medical Technicians, 133
National Board Dental Examinations, 9
National Board Examination (NBE), 97
National Board for Respiratory Care (NBRC), 82, 84
National Board of Chiropractic Examiners, 3
National Board of Examiners in Optometry, 27
National Board of Podiatric Examiners, 61
National Center for Competency Testing, 181, 183
National Certified Technician O.R., 181, 183
National Commission on Certification of Physician Assistants (NCCPA), 47-49
National Contact Lens Examiners (NCLE), 164, 166
National Council for Therapeutic Recreation Certification (NCTRC), 68, 69
National Credentialing Agency for Laboratory Personnel, 110, 113
National Federation of Licensed Practical Nurses, 139
National Highway Transportation Safety Administration, 133
National Institute of Occupational Safety and Health (NIOSH), 156, 158
National League for Nursing, 77, 138
National Registry of Emergency Medical Technicians (NREMT), 128, 130, 131, 133
National Therapeutic Recreation Society, 69
nervous system(s), 1, 53, 85, 89, 122

neuroanatomy, 41
neurological disorders, 89
neurological surgery, 53
neurology, 2, 3, 4, 40, 97, 150
neurophysiology, 28
neurosonographers, 122
neurosonography, 122, 124
nontraditional veterinary services, 98
North American Veterinary Licensing Exam (NAVLE), 97
nuclear medicine technologists, 105, 126, 147, 148, 149, 150, 174, 178
Nuclear Medicine Technology Certification Board, 149, 151
nuclear medicine technology, 149, 151, 173
nuclear pharmacy, 32
nurse supervisors, 72
nursing aides, 71, 72, 104, 105, 136
nursing assistants, 136
nursing care plans, 71
nursing homes, 13, 15, 16, 21, 33, 41, 46, 54, 60, 67, 68, 73, 75, 76, 79, 81, 83, 88, 90, 136, 137, 141, 143, 144
nutrition, 2-4, 13-17, 32, 72, 74, 96, 117, 137
nutritional counseling, 16
nutritional practices, 14
nutritional services, 13
nutritionists, 13-17

O

obstetric sonographers, 124
obstetrics, 47, 53, 55, 121, 123, 124, 137
Occupational Health and Safety Administration (OSHA), 155
Occupational Health and Safety Administration, 155
occupational health and safety inspectors, 153
occupational health and safety programs, 155
occupational health and safety specialists and technicians, 153-157, 159
Occupational Health and Safety Technologist (OHST), 156
Occupational Health and Safety Technologist, 156, 158
occupational therapist assistants, 21, 118, 172
Occupational therapists (OTs), 19
occupational therapists, 5, 19-23, 40, 43, 49, 66, 69, 77, 84, 91
occupational therapy, 22, 24
oncology, 32, 52, 97, 150
on-the-job training, 55, 156, 163, 169, 170, 181
open-heart surgery, 102
ophthalmic laboratory technicians, 162, 163, 165
ophthalmologists, vii, 26, 27, 28, 161, 163
ophthalmology, 53, 97
opticianry, 163, 165, 166
Opticians Association of America, 165
opticians, 26, 161-166
optometric services, 28
optometrists, 5, 11, 25, 26, 27, 28, 29, 58, 63, 91, 100, 161, 163
Optometry Admissions Test, 27
oral hygiene, 115, 116
oral motor problems, 86
orthodontists, 8
orthopedic surgery, 53
orthopedics, 2, 3, 4, 40, 46, 60, 62
orthotics, 60
orthotists, 165
outpatient rehabilitation programs, 23

P

pacemakers, 102

paramedics, 77, 127-133, 138
pathologists, 8, 85-91, 108, 110
pathology, 4, 47, 52, 55, 61, 86, 88, 91, 97, 117, 176
patient care, 75, 110, 124, 137, 142, 149, 176
patient counseling, 31
pediatric dentists, 8
pediatrics, 2, 40, 46, 47, 48, 53, 55, 60, 72, 75, 137
periodontists, 8
personal care facilities, 23, 43, 67, 69, 77, 138, 145
pharmaceutical companies, 31, 95
pharmacies, 32, 33, 34, 35, 36, 169, 171
pharmacists, 31, 32, 33, 34, 35, 36, 167, 168, 170, 171
pharmacology, 27, 34, 47, 55, 61, 117, 181
pharmacotherapy, 32
pharmacy aides, 32, 35, 36, 167, 171
Pharmacy College Admissions Test, 34
Pharmacy Technician Certification Board, 169, 172
pharmacy technician training programs, 170
pharmacy technicians, 32, 35, 167-171
pharmacy technology, 171
phlebotomists, 108
physical sciences, 149
physical therapist assistants, 118, 172
physical therapists (PTs), 5, 23, 39-43, 49, 62, 69, 77, 84, 91
physical therapy, 42, 43, 59
Physician Assistant-Certified (PA-C), 47
physician assistants(PAs), 45-49, 58, 77, 118, 131, 132
physiological optics, 28

physiology, 4, 9, 15, 47, 55, 67, 74, 82, 88, 96, 117, 124, 137, 141, 143, 145, 176, 181
pneumonia, 83
podiatric care, 62
podiatric medicine, 61, 62, 63
podiatrists, vii, 5, 11, 29, 58, 59, 60, 61, 62, 63, 100
police, 127, 128, 129, 132, 158
positron emission tomography (PET), 150
practical nursing, 136, 137, 138
premature infants, 80, 83, 89, 122
prescription drugs, 32, 35, 170
prescriptions, 7, 26, 34, 35, 161, 162, 167
preventive healthcare, 45, 51, 53
preventive medicine, 51, 52
primary care physicians, 53, 56
primary care providers, 53
primary medicine, 62
prisons, 14, 16, 46, 48
private agencies, 72
private practice, 2, 7-10, 14, 21, 26, 29, 41, 60, 88, 90, 94
private practices, 41, 60, 61, 93
problem solving, 20, 82, 86, 110
prosthetists, 165
prosthodontists, 8
psychiatric facilities, 68
psychiatric hospitals, 21
psychiatric nursing, 137
psychiatric rehabilitation, 65, 68
psychiatry, 47, 52, 53, 55, 75
psychologists, 11, 66, 86, 91
psychology, 4, 15, 27, 47, 55, 67, 74
public clinics, 48
public health clinics, 14, 46
public health departments, 75
public health, 4, 8, 14, 15, 16, 28, 46, 60, 73, 75, 95, 99, 116, 118
pulmonary medicine, 81

R

radiation therapists, 84, 151, 178
radiation, 2, 73, 105, 121, 125, 136, 147-150, 154, 174-176
radio waves, 121, 174
radioactivity, 147
radiobiology, 176
radiographers, 174, 175, 176
radiographs, 174
radiography, 117, 175-178
radiologic technologists and technicians, 105, 126, 147, 151, 173-177
radiologic technology, 147, 176
radiology, 52, 60, 61, 97, 174
radionuclides, 147, 148, 150
radiopharmaceuticals, 147, 148, 149, 150
reasoning abilities, 19, 65
recreation activities, 65, 66
recreational therapists, 23, 43, 65, 66, 67, 68, 69, 91
Registered Health Information Technicians (RHIT), 143, 144
Registered Health Information Technicians, 143
registered nurses (RNs), 17, 71-77, 84, 118, 131, 132, 135, 149, 175, 179
Registered Respiratory Therapist, 82
registered respiratory therapists (RRTs), 82
rehabilitation counselors, 23, 43, 69, 91
rehabilitation, 21, 23, 25, 41-43, 52, 66, 69, 71, 72, 76, 89, 91, 154
relaxation techniques, 66
residency, 28, 34, 48, 55, 56, 58, 61, 96, 97
residential care facilities, 15, 21, 66, 74, 136
residential facilities, 67, 68
respiratory ailments, 83
respiratory care treatments, 79

respiratory equipment, 79, 81
respiratory therapists, 23, 43, 77, 79, 80, 81, 82, 83, 105, 126, 151, 178
respiratory therapy clinics, 79, 83
respiratory therapy technicians, 79, 83, 182
retail optical stores, 27, 163
retail pharmacies, 32, 35, 167, 168, 170
retirement benefits, 11
retirement, 5, 8, 11, 63, 72, 132, 182

S

sanitation, 14, 94
scrubs, 179, 180
SDMS, 123
sign language, 86
skeletal system, 53
sleeping habits, 2
smoking cessation, 32
social sciences, 4, 22, 34, 47, 55, 96
social service agencies, 15, 16, 68, 74
social skills, 66
social workers, 40, 66, 86
Society of Diagnostic Medical Sonographers, 123, 126
Society of Vascular Technology, 106
solo practitioners, 8, 54, 59, 60, 94
sonographers, 102, 105, 121-126, 149, 151, 174, 178
sonography, 101, 105, 121-124, 126, 177
sound waves, 102, 121, 122
special education programs, 23, 66
speech problems, 85, 86
speech, 23, 27, 29, 40, 43, 49, 58, 85-91
speech-language pathologists, 23, 29, 40, 43, 49, 58, 85-90
speech-language pathology, 85
spinal column, 2
spinal cord injuries, 20
sports injuries, 2, 3

sports medicine, 40, 60
staff nurses, 71, 74
stress testing, 101
stress, 2, 4, 20, 65, 66, 81, 86, 104, 105, 127, 129, 136
strokes, 42, 72
substance abuse, 66, 67, 170
surgeons, 5, 8, 11, 26, 29, 51, 53, 54, 56, 63, 100, 135, 161, 179, 180, 181
surgery, 2, 4, 28, 46, 47, 48, 51-55, 60-62, 72, 75, 76, 80, 94, 95, 97, 101, 102, 150, 179-182
surgical procedures, 28, 48, 179, 181, 182
surgical technologists, 138, 172, 179-182
surgicenters, 72, 76, 137
swallowing disorders, 86

T

telemedicine, 48
therapeutic recreation, 65-68
therapeutic services, 19, 23, 39, 42
therapy services, 22, 42, 89
thermography, 3
transesophageal echocardiography, 103
transfusions, 107
transmissible diseases, 94
trauma, 42, 87, 89, 128, 130
treatment plans, 39, 72, 141

U

U.S. Air Force, 98
U.S. Armed Forces, 110, 175
U.S. Army, 98
U.S. Department of Agriculture, 95
U.S. Department of Veterans Affairs, 15, 46, 54, 60, 109

U.S. Public Health Service, 60, 98, 109
ultra- sound instrumentation, 102
ultrasonics, 116
ultrasonography, 121
urology, 56

V

vascular sonographers, 102
vascular technologists, 102, 104, 105
vascular technology, 101, 104-106, 122
ventilators, 80
veterinarians, 5, 11, 29, 58, 63, 93-100
Veterinary College Admission Test (VCAT), 96
veterinary education, 96, 100
veterinary medical colleges, 95, 96, 97
veterinary medicine, 93, 95, 97, 100
veterinary services, 94, 98
veterinary technologists, 100, 112
viral infections, 87
vision care, 25, 26, 28, 164
vision problems, 25, 28
vision therapy, 25, 26, 28
visual science, 28
voice quality problems, 85

W

well-being, 65, 66
wellness programs, 14
work environments, 72, 153
work skills, 19
workplaces, 87, 153, 154, 155

X

x rays, 2, 7, 45, 60, 62, 115, 141, 173, 174